英語総合教材

English for Nursing Students

看護系学生のための総合英語

Marilyn W. Edmunds
Paul Price
大瀧祥子
引地岳雄

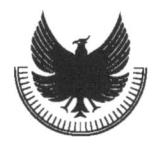

NAN'UN-DO

English for Nursing Students
by
Marilyn W. Edmunds
Paul Price
Sachiko Ohtaki
Takeo Hikichi
© 1998 All Rights Reserved

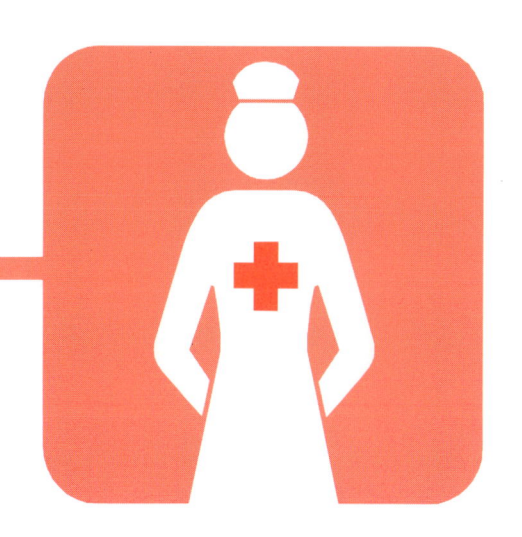

はしがき

　本書は、看護学の現場からの新鮮かつわかりやすい読み物と会話、それを基にした役に立つ練習問題、楽しみながら自然に英語で話せるLET'S TALKから成っています。看護系学生が興味を持ちながら、将来必要な英語の4技能を無理なく身につけることができるように工夫してあります。

　＜本書の構成＞
1. Reading Text
　　現在、米国の医系大学Family Nurse Practitioner科の主任教授であるDr. Marilyn W. Edmunds が日本の学生のために書き下ろしたものです。平易な英語と共に丁寧な注釈をつけましたから、無理なく看護の基本を理解することができます。内容を理解した後、是非テープを利用して音読の練習をし、速読速解を心がけて、最後は音声のみで理解できるようにしてください。

- **Vocabulary:** 看護系学生が使用するであろう語彙を選んであります。繰り返し発音して身につけてください。
- **Questions & Answers:** 段階をおって本文の理解を確認するようにしてあります。最後に自分で質問を作って、クラスの皆で答えるようにしてみましょう。
- **Grammar & Usage:** すでに身につけている基本的な文法を再確認するためのものです。

2. Dialogue
- **Dialogue A:** Dr. Edmundsの書き下ろしたものです。実際ナースが遭遇しそうな会話になっています。CDをよく聴いて内容把握の後、CDの音声のみで理解できるようにしてください。
- **Dialogue B:** Dr. Edmundsの書き下ろしを学生が練習しやすいように一部変えたものです。また、右端に談話構成が書いてあります。英文をかくして構成だけ見て言えるようにするのもよい練

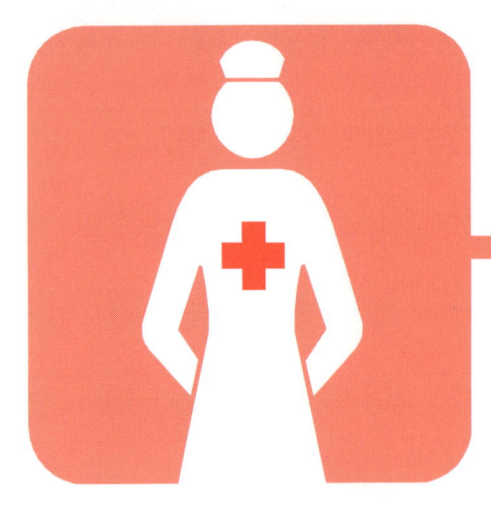

習です。
- **True or False:** Dialogue Aの内容についての簡単なセンテンスを聞き取り、判断する練習です。書き取りに使用するのもよいでしょう。
- **Dialogue Practice:** Dialogue Bの基本的な文型を練習した後、パートナーと練習します。
- **Vocabulary:** 看護系学生が使用するであろう語彙を選んであげてあります。繰り返し発音して身につけてください。

3. LET'S TALK

看護系学生に必要な語彙を、将来ありうる場面で楽しく練習できるようになっています。従来の医系語学教材に欠けていると思われるもので、コミュニケーション能力開発をめざすものです。

巻末に、2、3で使用した表現をまとめたUseful Expressionsを載せました。活用してください。

本書は4人の共同作業でできました。上記のDr. Edmundsは読み物とDialogueの書き下ろしを、Paul Price氏はLET'S TALKの制作と英文の添削を、引地岳雄氏は読み物の注釈と添削、大瀧は企画編集と練習問題その他を担当いたしました。

本書出版にあたってはたくさんの方々の御協力をいただきました。特にDr. Edmundsの英文執筆に際して御助力いただいたMs. Christy Crowther, MSに深く感謝します。また、さし絵を描いていただいた前田印刷の作田和美さん、金沢医科大学付属看護専門学校生徒の坂井美和さん、道下由香さん、そして最後に、本書出版に際して種々ご尽力くださった南雲堂編集長の青木泰祐氏、および大井理江子さんに心から感謝いたします。

1998年4月　　　　大瀧祥子

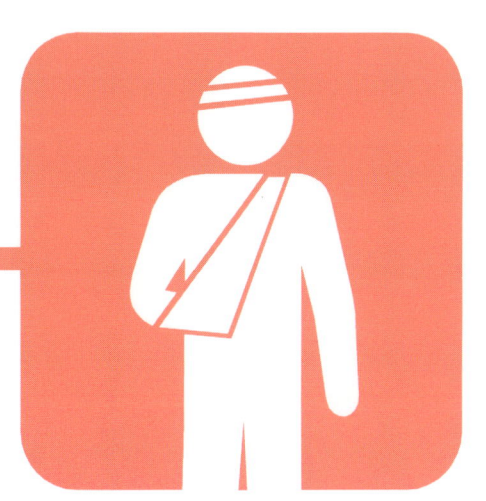

CONTENTS

Chapter 1   **WHAT IS A NURSE?** ················ 7
    ——看護とは
       1. What Is a Nurse?
       2. What Kind of Things Do Nurses Do?
       3. LET'S TALK: Things That Nurses Do

Chapter 2   **THE HISTORY OF NURSING** ················ 15
    ——看護の歴史
       1. How Did Nursing Begin?
       2. Nightingale's Advice Is Still Important Today
       3. LET'S TALK: Describing Medical Instruments

Chapter 3   **PATIENT-NURSE RELATIONSHIP** ················ 23
    ——患者と看護師の関係
       1. The Nurse Has a Special Relationship with the Patient
       2. The Patient Needs Me
       3. LET'S TALK: Asking for Personal Details

Chapter 4   **COMMUNICATION WITH A PATIENT** ················ 31
    ——患者とのコミュニケーション
       1. Good Communication with a Patient Is Important
       2. Thank You for Talking to Me
       3. LET'S TALK: Listening to and Sympathizing with the Patient

Chapter 5   **INTERCULTURAL COMMUNICATION WITH A PATIENT** ······ 39
    ——患者との異文化コミュニケーション
       1. How Can Culture Cause Problems?
       2. Something Special for Me
       3. LET'S TALK: Avoiding and Solving Difficulties

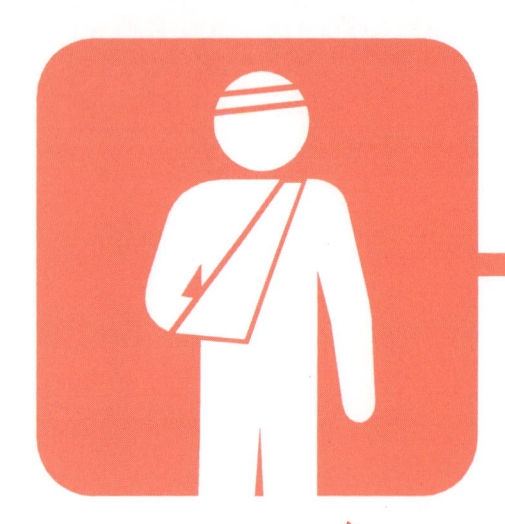

Chapter 6   DOCTOR-NURSE RELATIONSHIP ……………… 47
——医師と看護師の関係
 1. Nurses Work Closely with Doctors
 2. That's Important Information
 3. LET'S TALK: The Nurse Seeks Advice from the Doctor

Chapter 7   RELATED PROFESSIONALS ………………… 55
——関連のある職種の人達
 1. Nurses Work with Related Professionals
 2. We Work as Part of the Health Care Team
 3. LET'S TALK: Consulting a Specialist

Chapter 8   NURSES AND THE HOSPITAL …………………… 63
——看護師と病院
 1. The Work Nurses Do Depends on the Type of Hospital
 2. So Busy Tonight
 3. LET'S TALK: Working in the Hospital

Chapter 9   NURSES IN THE COMMUNITY ………………… 71
——地域における看護師
 1. Nurses Work Outside the Hospital
 2. To Prevent You from Getting Injured
 3. LET'S TALK: The Nurse Is Teaching Outside the Hospital

Chapter 10   NURSING IN THE FUTURE ……………………… 79
——未来の看護
 1. How Will Nursing Change in the Future?
 2. Nursing on the Internet
 3. LET'S TALK: What Type of Nurse Do You Want to Be?

Chapter 1

WHAT IS A NURSE?

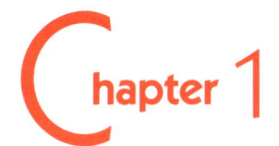

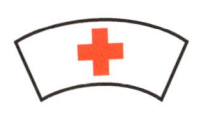

1. What Is a Nurse?

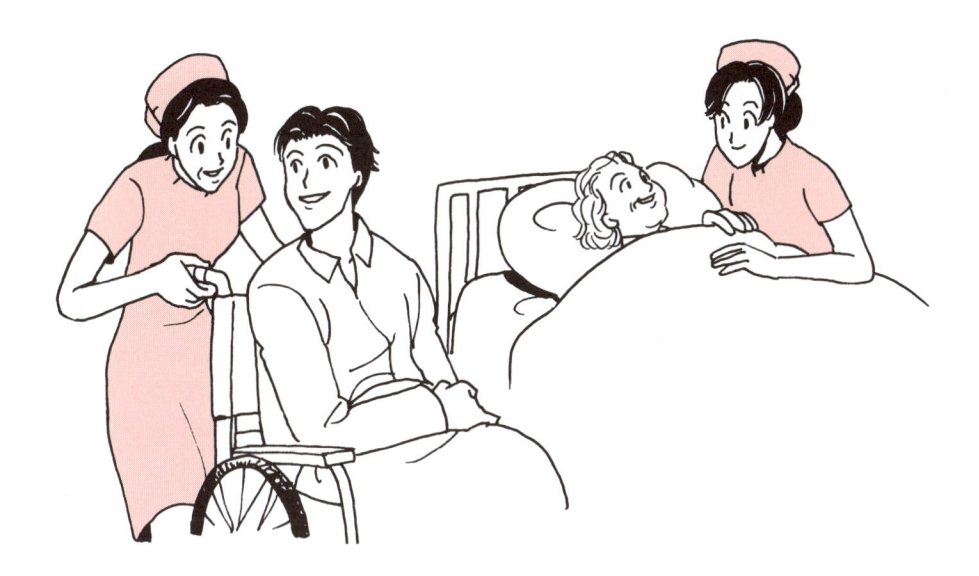

Nursing is a process to assist people in improving their health. Nurses primarily deal with two groups of people: the sick, who need someone to help them when they cannot care for themselves, and the well, who need education to help them stay well. Nursing focuses on "caring" for patients, not "curing" them.

The nursing process guides the action of nurses. First, the nurse assesses the patient's problem. Because one's health is based upon many things, nurses must make a total or "holistic" assessment. This requires them to consider not only physical problems, but also mental, spiritual, cultural, financial, or social factors that may be influencing the patient. Once they understand the patient's problems, nurses help make a plan for solving the problems. Next, the nurse works with the patient to carry out the plan. This may require working with other health care providers, or the patient's family, or using the resources in the community. Finally, the nurse must evaluate whether the problem is solved or not. Many problems require work over a long time. Thus, good communication skills and a trusting relationship between nurse and patient are very important.

Notes: 看護は人々の健康増進を助ける一過程だが、その内容は…？
process「過程」ある手順をふむ過程または方法 **assist people in** …「人々が…するのを助ける」 **primarily**「本来」 **the sick**「病人」the＋形容詞は〈…な人々〉を意味する **care for** …「…を看護する」 **the well**「健康な人々」 **stay well**「健康なままでいる、健康を維持する」 **focus(es) on** …「…することに焦点をしぼる、…することに専念する」 **nursing process**「看護過程」事前評価、看護計画、実践、事後評価と進む看護の道筋 **problem**「問題」だが、ここでは病気や症状のこと **holistic**「全体論的」次の文に説明がある **health care providers**「ヘルスケア提供者、医療関係者」 **carry out** …「…を実行する」 **resources**「（人的、物的）資源」 **trusting relationship**「信頼関係」

✚ Vocabulary

Match the similar expressions.

1. well   (   )   a. of the body
2. sick   (   )   b. of the mind
3. assess   (   )   c. healthy
4. physical (   )   d. ill
5. mental   (   )   e. evaluate

1. WHAT IS A NURSE?

✚ Questions & Answers

> **1. 2.** Choose the best answer.
> **3. 4.** Answer in English.
> **5.** Make your own question.

1. What does nursing focus on?
   a. caring for patients   b. curing patients
   c. educating patients

2. What do nurses first do to solve patients' problems?
   a. They carry out a plan.   b. They make an assessment.
   c. They make a plan.

3. What factors may influence patients?
   _____
   _____

4. What do nurses finally do to solve patients' problems?
   _____
   _____

5. Your question _____
   _____
   Answer _____

✚ Grammar & Usage

> Fill in each blank with one word from the list below. Use each of them only once.

[once   because   when   although   till]

1. (   ) you cannot sleep well, this medicine will help you rest.
2. Don't worry. I will stay here (   ) you fall asleep.
3. (   ) you start a plan, you should not change it.
4. (   ) it was difficult to carry out the plan by herself, Beth had to ask for help.
5. (   ) Tom had a hearing problem, he managed to graduate at the top of his class.

2. What Kind of Things Do Nurses Do?

Dialogue A 〈A: Girl　B: Nurse〉

看護師志望の少女が知り合いのNurseに出会って…。

A: Do nurses just do what the doctor tells them to do?

B: No. We do work with doctors. But there are many things only nurses do to help patients get well.

A: What kind of things do nurses do?

B: Nurses spend a lot of time with patients. Through information about their concerns and problems, we can help decide what will be most helpful to them in their recovery.

A: But you mostly work with sick people in the hospital, don't you? You give them baths and make them take medicine, right?

B: Well, we do all those things. However, we also teach people in schools or offices about risks to their health and how to stay well.

A: Maybe I'll be a nurse when I grow up. I would like to help people get better when they are sick.

Notes:　**concern**「懸念、心配」　**medicine**「薬」、「医学」の意味もある　**risk**「危険性、おそれ」

Dialogue B 〈A: Nurse　B: Mr. Brown〉

職場のNurseが工場で働くBrownさんに…。

A: Hi. It looks like your wrist is hurting you. — 間接的な質問

B: Yes. It hurts a lot. — 答え

A: Have you sprained it? — 直接的な質問

B: I'm not sure. In the morning it's fine. But by the time I leave it's pretty swollen. And at night it hurts a lot. — 答え

A: Well, maybe you should give it a rest every couple of hours and put an ice pack on it. — 示唆

B: Good idea. Thanks a lot. — 同意、感謝

Notes:　**wrist**「手首」(p.90の図参照)　**sprain**「(足首、手首などを)くじく、捻挫する」
by the time ～「～までには」　**every couple of hours**「2時間毎に」

1. WHAT IS A NURSE?

✚ True or False (Dialogue A)

> Listen and write what you hear. Then circle T (true) or F (false).

1. _____ T / F
2. _____ T / F
3. _____ T / F
4. _____ T / F
5. _____ T / F

✚ Dialogue Practice (Dialogue B)

> **1.** Substitute the words shown below or follow the instructions.

▶ sentence: **It looks like your wrist is hurting you.**

（p.90の図参照）

1. your foot → _____
2. your knee → _____
3. your shoulder → _____
4. you are getting well → _____

▶ sentence: **Have you sprained it?**

1. he → _____
2. break → _____
3. 肯定文 → _____
4. 否定文 → _____

> **2.** Practice the dialogue.

✚ Vocabulary (Dialogues A and B)

> Choose the word that means the same as the expression on the right, as it is used in the text.

1. medicine ( )   a. damage by sudden twisting
2. hurt   ( )   b. bigger than normal
3. wrist   ( )   c. substance used for treating disease
4. sprain   ( )   d. cause pain
5. swollen   ( )   e. the joint between the hand and the arm

3. LET'S TALK: Things That Nurses Do

✚ What do nurses do?

1. Nurseのすることをできるだけ書き出してみましょう。

2. 次にNurseのすることの例があります。関係のある絵の番号を書き入れましょう。

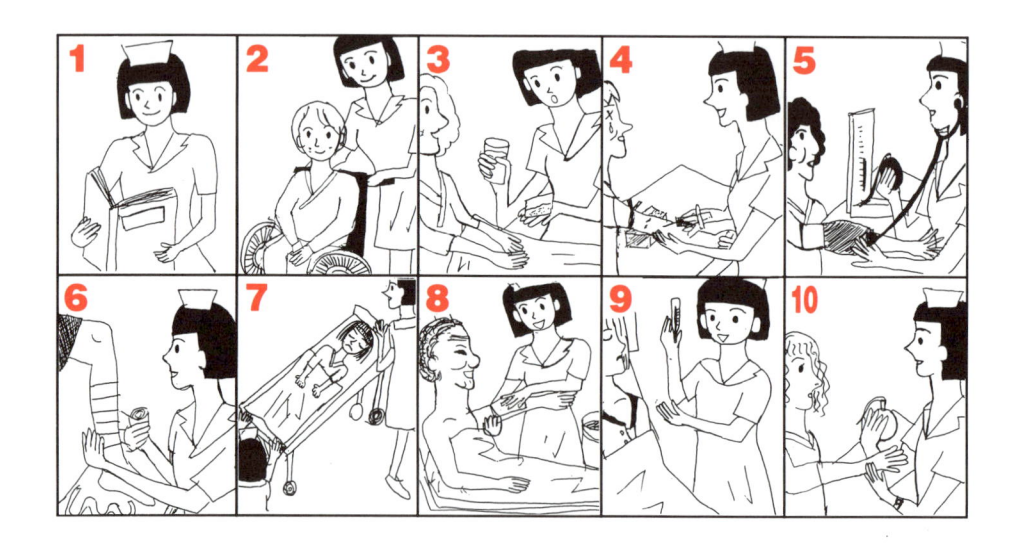

    - checking the blood pressure (　)
    - taking the temperature (　)
    - giving medicine (　)　　　• changing bandages (　)
    - giving a bed-bath (　)　　• looking at a chart (　)
    - giving an injection (　)　　• taking the pulse (　)
    - pushing a person in a wheelchair (　)
    - carrying a patient on a stretcher (　)

3. CDを聴いて発音しましょう。

1. WHAT IS A NURSE?

✚ What are the nurses doing? (Pair Work)

1. よく似ているけれど少しずつちがう絵A，Bがあります。あなたとパートナーとどちらかちがう絵を選びましょう。
2. 選んだ絵の10人の患者とその周りの様子を英語でメモしましょう。
3. 例にならって各々の絵の患者とnurseの様子の違いについてパートナーと交互に話し合いましょう。

[例]

> A: A big nurse is feeding a patient. The patient's lying in bed. She has black hair.
> B: In my picture, a small nurse is carrying food to a patient. The patient's young and is sitting up in bed. Another nurse is….
> A: In my picture….

4. あなたの絵とパートナーの絵との違いをメモしてみましょう。

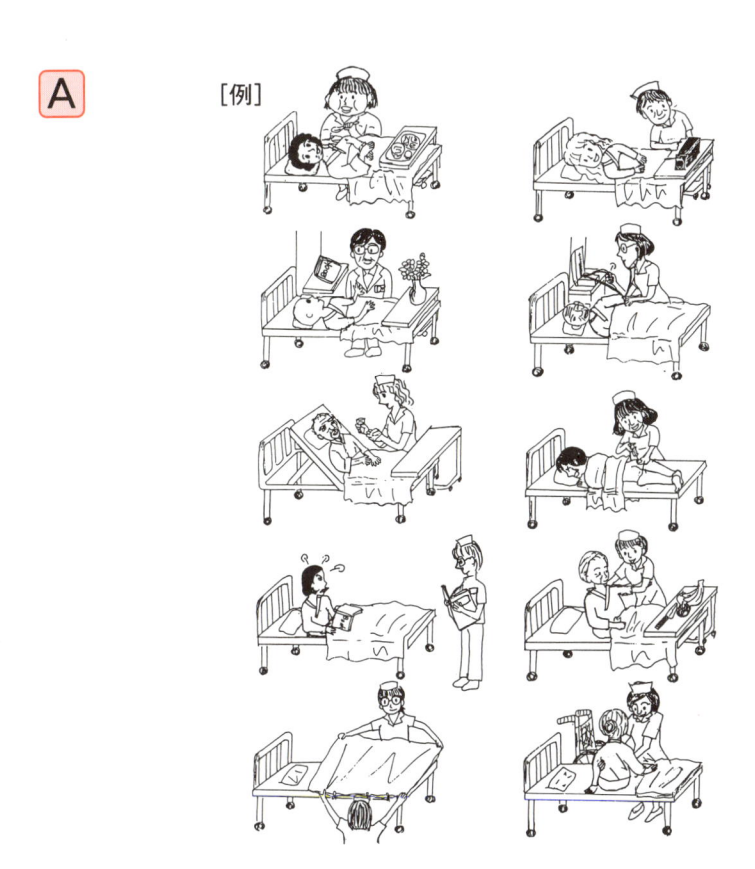

A   [例]

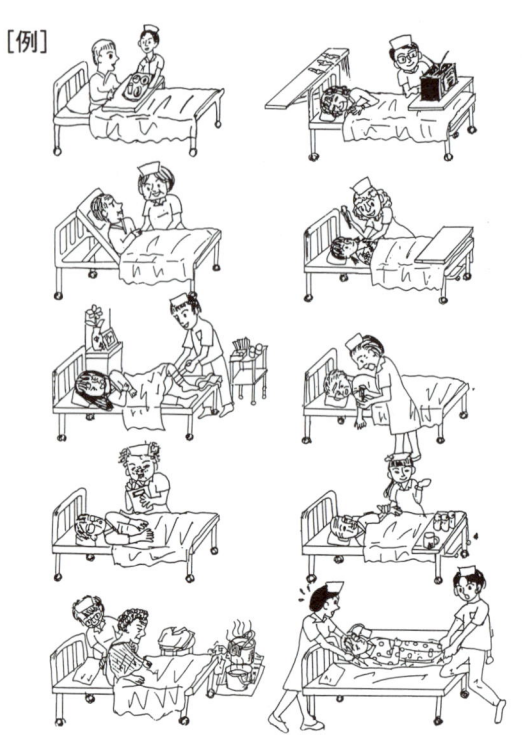

B

✚ Dialogue Practice

1. 次のB～Hについて、Aにならって過去形を書きましょう。

    A. to check your blood pressure   <u> checked </u>
    B. to switch on the TV   _____
    C. to make the bed   _____
    D. to take some medicine   _____
    E. to examine your foot   _____
    F. to have an injection   _____
    G. to feed a baby   _____
    H. to take your pulse   _____

2. 次の例のイタリックの部分をかえて、パートナーとdialogueをしてみましょう。（一方は上記のA～D、他方はE～Hを使用）

[例] A: When was the last time you *went to the hospital*?
      B: *One week ago*.

[参考] two days ago／last week／last year／yesterday／last night／this morning／never／I don't remember

Chapter 2

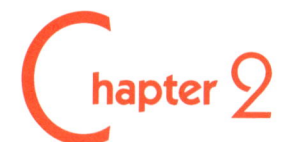

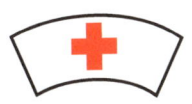

THE HISTORY OF NURSING

1. How Did Nursing Begin?

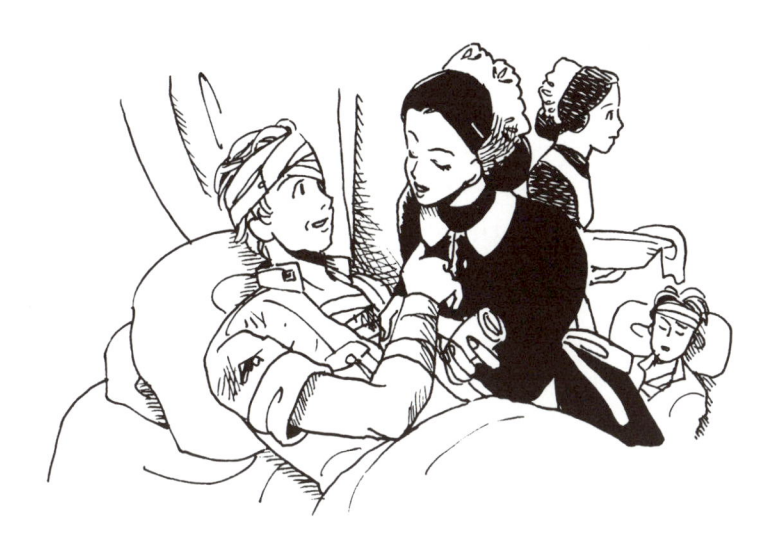

In the past, most people died when they became sick or were injured. Over time, information about the body and how to heal it grew from watching what happened to soldiers injured in battle. The discovery of such information led to advances in anesthesia, surgery and pharmacology and helped more patients stay alive. Thus, more and more nurses became necessary to care for the sick who did not die.

There have always been kind men and women who tried to care for the injured and diseased. However, it was not until the Crimean War of the 1850's that nursing as we know it began. Under the leadership of a wealthy, well-educated Englishwoman,

Florence Nightingale, women were found and given lessons in how to care for injured soldiers. The first efforts of nurses were not appreciated by the military surgeons and physicians with whom they worked. However, it was clear that their efforts saved hundreds of soldiers' lives.

Over the last 90 years, formal educational programs have slowly developed in hospitals and then in universities to train nurses in scientific knowledge. Physicians have grown to depend on nurses to do many things for the patient. The nurse has become a respectable member of a team that helps care for patients.

Notes: 昔は、病気になったりけがをしたりすると、ほとんどの人が死んだ。 **Over time**「時が経つにつれて」 **heal**「(傷、痛みなどを) いやす、なおす」 *cf.* **cure**「治療する、なおす」 **led to ...** ＜ lead to ...「…を引き起こす」 **anesthesia**「麻酔」 **surgery**「外科、手術」 **pharmacology**「薬理学」 **stay alive**「生きたままでいる、生命を維持する」 **the injured and diseased**「けが人や病人」injureは他動詞で「傷つける」受身形で「怪我をする」 **it was not until ... that** ～「…になってようやく～した」 **the Crimean** [kraimíːən] **War**「クリミア戦争」(1853-56) ロシアがトルコ領内のギリシア正教徒保護を名目にバルカン半島に侵攻。トルコ、英、仏、サルジニャの連合軍が勝利して、ロシアの南下政策は失敗。 **nursing as we know it**「今日私たちが知っているような看護」 **well-educated**「高度な教育を受けた」 **were not appreciated**「正当に評価されなかった」 **Over the last 90 years**「この90年間に」 **formal educational programs**「正規の教育課程」 **have grown to depend on ... to** ～「…が～するのを当てにするようになってきた」 **respectable**「尊敬すべき、りっぱな」

✚ Vocabulary

Match the similar expressions.

1. injure   (　)   a. operation
2. anesthesia   (　)   b. study of drugs
3. surgery   (　)   c. doctor
4. pharmacology (　)   d. being unable to feel pain
5. physician   (　)   e. hurt

2. THE HISTORY OF NURSING

➕ Questions & Answers

> 1. 2. Choose the best answer.
> 3. 4. Answer in English.
> 5. Make your own question.

1. How was information gained about the body?
   a. from fighting in battles   b. from touching the body
   c. from watching the injured

2. Where was Florence Nightingale from?
   a. the U. S. A.   b. England   c. Crimea

3. When did nursing as we know it begin?
   _____
   _____

4. What did doctors in Nightingale's days think about nurses?
   _____
   _____

5. Your question _____
   _____
   Answer _____

➕ Grammar & Usage

> Fill in each blank with one word from the list below. Use each of them only once.

[which   who   whom   whose   where]

1. There were a lot of injured soldiers (   ) needed medical care.
2. Nursing students study in hospitals (   ) doctors and nurses train them.
3. The physician with (   ) the nurse worked in the hospital lived near her apartment.
4. The nurse gave the physician a lot of information (   ) would be very useful for treating the patient.
5. Who will care for the child (   ) mother is working in the hospital?

2. Nightingale's Advice Is Still Important Today

Dialogue A ⟨A: Florence Nightingale   B: Young woman⟩

Nightingale が若い女性に出会って…。

A: I'm looking for strong, practical women who are not afraid to work.

B: I don't know what to do for someone who is sick or injured.

A: I believe there are many things we can do.

B: I think it would be very hard work. Is it dangerous?

A: No. We won't be on the battlefield. We'll have the injured brought to us.

B: I feel so sorry for the soldiers when they are injured. I think I'd like to help them.

A: We can help keep them clean. And we can give them nourishing food. We can wrap their injuries. And we can assist the physicians.

B: I could do all those things.

Notes: look for ~「~を探す」   battlefield「戦場」   nourishing「滋養になる」

Dialogue B ⟨A and B: Two Nursing Students⟩

二人の看護学生が Nightingale の映画を見終わって…。

A: You know, many of Florence Nightingale's ideas and her procedures are still important today.	意見
B: That's true! Like, it's important to observe the patient. Closely.	同意、理由、例
A: And we must write down what the patient does.	他の例
B: And also we've to write down what we do.	他の例
A: Yes. Keeping an accurate record is vital.	要約、結論
B: Definitely!	同意

Notes: procedure「処置」   accurate「正確な」   vital ＜ vive(F.)「命の」「きわめて大切な」
vital signs「生命徴候」(脈拍、体温など)   definitely「まったく（そのとおり）」

2. THE HISTORY OF NURSING

🔴 True or False (Dialogue A)   (CD 11)

> Listen and write what you hear. Then circle T (true) or F (false).

1. _____ T / F
2. _____ T / F
3. _____ T / F
4. _____ T / F
5. _____ T / F

🔴 Dialogue Practice (Dialogue B)

> **1.** Substitute the words shown below or follow the instructions.

▶ sentence: **It's important to observe the patient.**
   1. necessary → _____
   2. vital → _____
   3. listen to → _____
   4. 過去形 → _____

▶ sentence: We must write down **what the patient does.**
   1. we → _____
   2. say → _____
   3. how, feel → _____
   4. 過去形 → _____

> **2.** Practice the dialogue.

🔴 Vocabulary (Dialogues A and B)   (CD 13)

> Choose the word that means the same as the expression on the right, as it is used in the text.

1. injury   (   )   a. written statement of facts
2. wrap   (   )   b. actions necessary for doing something
3. procedure   (   )   c. watch carefully
4. observe   (   )   d. damage to a living thing
5. record   (   )   e. cover

3. LET'S TALK: Describing Medical Instruments

🏥 Vocabulary

1. CDを聴いて単語を発音しましょう。

- ambulance   • microscope   • spectacles   • syringe
- sphygmomanometer   • stethoscope   • thermometer

ヒント： **micro-** = small   **therm-** = temperature   **spect-** = to see
sphygmo- = pulse   **manometer** = pressure measure

2. 単語をその絵の下に書きましょう。

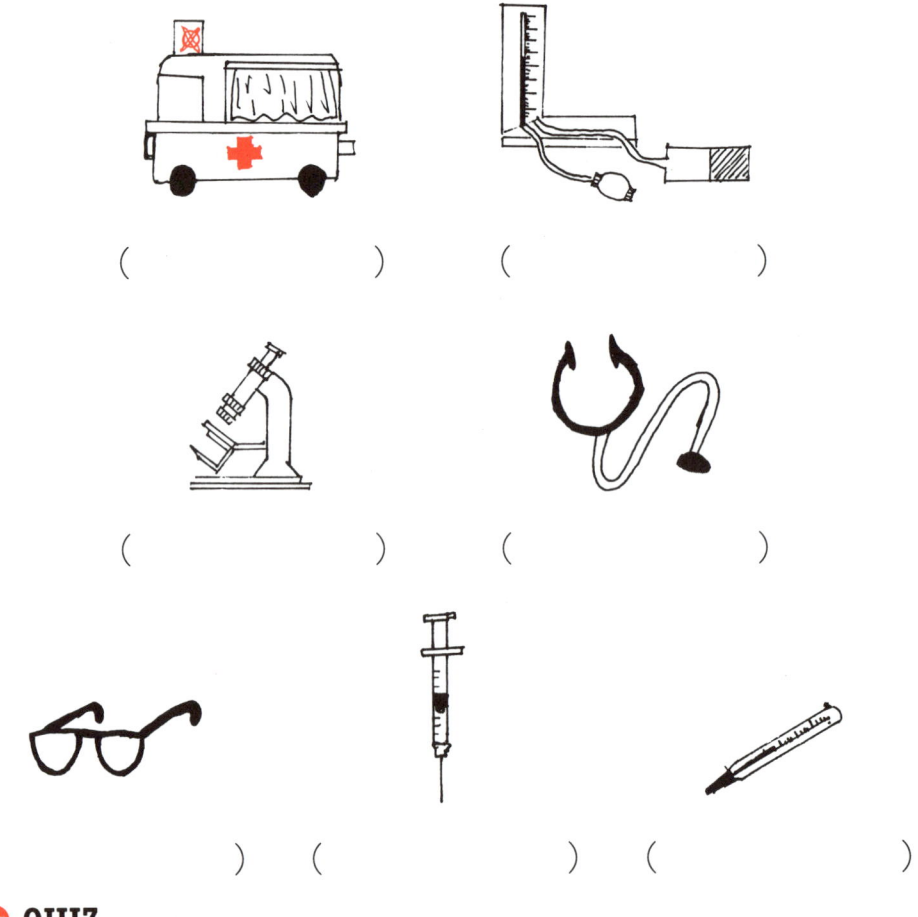

(   )   (   )

(   )   (   )

(   )   (   )   (   )

🏥 QUIZ

1. CDを聴いて年号を発音しましょう。

1998   1850   1341   1722   1668

2. THE HISTORY OF NURSING

🔊 16　2．次の質問のCDをよく聴いて空所に単語を入れましょう。いつ頃のことかクイズで当ててみましょう。年号を発音しましょう。

1. When was the first (　　　　　　) made?
   1290　　　1390　　　1490　　　1590
2. When was the first (　　　　　　) made?
   1416　　　1616　　　1816　　　1916
3. When was the first (　　　　　　) made?
   1680　　　1780　　　1880　　　1980
4. When were (　　　　　　) invented?
   1085　　　1285　　　1485　　　1685
5. When was the first (　　　　　　) made?
   1653　　　1753　　　1853　　　1953
6. When was the first (　　　　　　) invented?
   1292　　　1492　　　1592　　　1892
7. When was the first (　　　　　　) introduced?
   1287　　　1487　　　1687　　　1887
8. When was (　　　　　　) discovered?
   1828　　　1878　　　1928　　　1978
9. When were (　　　　　　) discovered?
   1805　　　1850　　　1895　　　1940

🔊 17　✚ **DESCRIPTIONS**

1．物をどう説明するかの練習です。CDを聴いて発音しましょう。

1. *It's*　　　　　a machine.
   　　　　　　　a tool.
   　　　　　　　a drug.
2. *It's made of*　wood.
   　　　　　　　plastic.
   　　　　　　　metal.
   　　　　　　　glass.
3. *It's used for*　eating.
   　　　　　　　measuring temperature.
   　　　　　　　lowering blood pressure.
   　　　　　　　looking at small objects.
   　　　　　　　cutting.

2. CDをよく聴いて **Vocabulary**（p.20）の絵のうちのどれについて言っているのか考え、その単語を書きましょう。

1. _____ 2. _____ 3. _____ 4. _____
5. _____ 6. _____ 7. _____

3. 次の絵のものを説明してみましょう。

① ② ③

4. Pair Work

パートナーに見えないようになにか絵を描いてみましょう。描いた絵をパートナーに説明してみましょう。パートナーはその絵が何かあてましょう。交代して絵を描いて説明しましょう。

描くものの例（CDをよく聴いて発音してみましょう）
- bed • glove • bowl • needle（針） • chair
- sink（台所の流し） • face mask • aspirin
- wheelchair（車椅子） • pacemaker • trolley
- crutch（松葉杖）

あなたの絵

Chapter 3

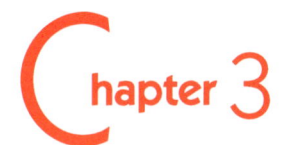

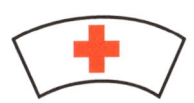

PATIENT-NURSE RELATIONSHIP

1. The Nurse Has a Special Relationship with the Patient

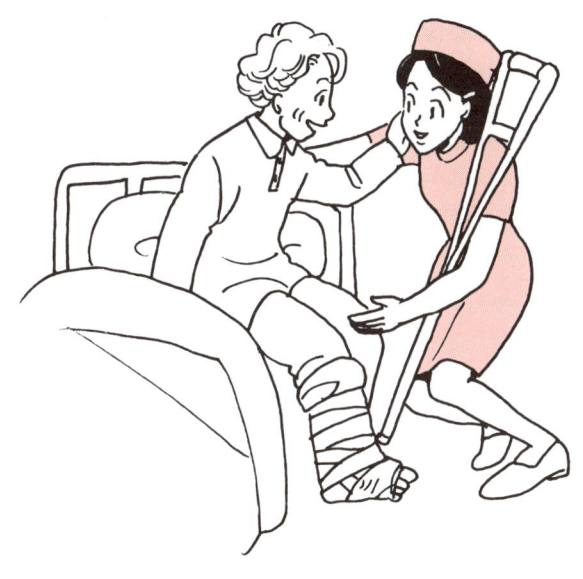

The nurse working with a patient has a very special relationship with him or her. The nurse learns to value each different individual and to help that person do things to get well. This can only happen when the nurse has a caring attitude and has the patient's cooperation in getting well. The patient does not "belong to" the nurse and the nurse cannot make the patient do things he or she does not want to do.

Some patients do things that harm their health: they may smoke, take drugs, or drink too much alcohol. Some patients do not show good judgment: they may wait until they are very ill, or until their children have many serious symptoms before seeking help. If the nurse is impatient or critical of the patient, it is difficult to have a trusting relationship between nurse and patient.

15 Scientific knowledge about the body helps nurses decide what to do. Nurses must also learn to understand patients. They need to learn about the things that are important to patients. It is only through learning this information that a helpful relationship may develop.

Notes: 患者さんを相手に働く看護師は（患者さんと）特別な関係をもつ。 **value each different individual**「さまざまな人ひとりひとりを尊重する」 **caring attitude**「思いやる態度」 **… cooperation in getting well**「回復にあたって…の協力」 **does not "belong to" …**「…にいわゆる "所属する" のではない、…のいわゆる "所有物" ではない」 **take drugs**「麻薬を常用する」 **show good judgment**「すぐれた判断力を示す」 **symptom**「症状（患者の言う）」 *cf.* sign「徴候（医師がみつける）」 **critical of …**「…に批判的」 **It is only through … that ~**（強調構文）「～は、…を通じてだけだ」 **helpful relationship**「有益な関係」

21 ✚ Vocabulary

Match the similar expressions.

1. relationship (　)　　a. manner of feeling and behaving
2. attitude　　(　)　　b. damage
3. cooperation (　)　　c. connection
4. harm　　　 (　)　　d. change in body which shows
5. symptom　 (　)　　　　disease
　　　　　　　　　　　 e. working together for a shared
　　　　　　　　　　　　　purpose

3. PATIENT-NURSE RELATIONSHIPS

✚ Questions & Answers

> **1. 2.** Choose the best answer.
> **3. 4.** Answer in English.
> **5.** Make your own question.

1. What attitude should a nurse have towards a patient?
   a. caring attitude   b. critical attitude
   c. determined attitude

2. What kind of relationship should a nurse have with a patient?
   a. a friendly relationship   b. a lifelong relationship
   c. a trusting relationship

3. What habits will harm your health?
   _____

4. What attitudes will make it difficult for the nurse to have a good relationship with the patient?
   _____

5. Your question _____
   _____
   Answer _____

✚ Grammar & Usage

> Fill in each blank with one word from the list below. Use each of them only once.

[before   by the time   if   until   when]

1. (   ) you listen to patients carefully, you will see what their problems are.
2. The mother fainted (   ) she heard the sad news.
3. I am sure you will have gotten well (   ) your father returns from the U.S.A.
4. After the operation the patient slept deeply (   ) the anesthetist woke him up.
5. It will not be long (   ) Pat comes back from the hospital.

2. The Patient Needs Me

Dialogue A 〈A: Mother   B: Nurse〉

妊婦が息せき切って入ってきて…。

A: (Crying) My baby is going to be born. Help me! Help me!

B: Mrs. Edwards, it's time for you to put on this gown.

A: Do you think the baby will come soon?

B: As soon as you get into bed, we will see when the baby is ready to come.

A: The doctor told me to come to the hospital when my contractions were five minutes apart.

B: Do you have any other symptoms?

A: I also feel a little nauseated. Is this normal?

B: Yes. Sometimes just before the baby is born, you feel nauseated.

A: Now I feel like I need to push.

B: Wait, I will go and get the doctor.

Notes: **contraction**「収縮」   **nauseated**「吐き気がする」   **push**「(分娩時に)息む」

Dialogue B 〈A: Mr. Sands   B: Nurse〉

糖尿病 (diabetes) のSands氏 (60才後半) が看護師と…。

A: I've had diabetes for a long long time. Now the doctor says I must take insulin shots.	何が起こっているか知りたい
B: Yes, your diabetes is getting a little worse. That's normal as you get older.	説明
A: I had to go to the toilet about 6 times last night.	訴え
B: The insulin will help you.	安心させる
A: Will I have to inject it myself? Maybe I won't be able to see the syringe properly.	不安
B: Don't worry about that. We'll give it to you for now.	安心させる

Notes: **insulin**「インスリン (血液中の炭水化物を調節するホルモン、糖尿病の特効薬)」   **shot**「注射」   **inject**「注射する」   **syringe**「注射器」   **properly**「正しく」

3. PATIENT-NURSE RELATIONSHIPS

🞣 True or False (Dialogue A)

Listen and write what you hear. Then circle T (true) or F (false).

1. _____ T / F
2. _____ T / F
3. _____ T / F
4. _____ T / F
5. _____ T / F

🞣 Dialogue Practice (Dialogue B)

1. Substitute the words shown below or follow the instructions.

▶ sentence: **I've had diabetes for a long time.**
   1. he → _____
   2. be ill → _____
   3. How long, you → _____

▶ sentence: **I had to go to the toilet about 6 times last night.**
   1. 現在形 → _____
   2. to take medicine after each meal → _____
   3. 疑問文 (you) → _____

▶ sentence: **Will I have to inject it myself?**
   1. you → _____
   2. to have surgery → _____
   3. 肯定文 → _____

2. Practice the dialogue.

🞣 Vocabulary (Dialogues A and B)

Choose the word that means the same as the expression on the right, as it is used in the text.

1. contraction   (   )   a. substance which controls blood sugar level
2. nauseated   (   )   b. a sort of pipe used for injections
3. diabetes   (   )   c. very strong tightening of the muscles
4. insulin   (   )   d. disease related to blood sugar level
5. syringe   (   )   e. feeling sick and wanting to vomit

3. LET'S TALK: Asking for Personal Details

✚ Dialogue Practice A

1．下記のDialogueを読んで、Nurseの質問を自分でつくってみましょう。
2．CDを聴いて確かめましょう。
3．パートナーと練習してみましょう。

Dialogue ⟨A: Nurse B: Mrs.Patella⟩

Mrs. Patella 入院1日目の朝に…。

A: Good morning. I'm Nurse Brown. _____?
B: Patella. Pelvis Patella.
A: _____?
B: Patella. P-a-t-e-l-l-a.
A: OK. Ms. Patella, I'd like to ask you a few questions about your personal details.
B: OK.
A: _____?
B: 12 Rib Street, Abdomen City.
A: _____?
B: April 4, 1965.
A: _____?
B: Yes. Two. A boy and a girl.

✚ Pair Work
[Step 1]

Mrs. Patellaのかわりに患者の役になる人物を自分で創って空欄をうめましょう。

Surname:		Given Name:	
Address:			
Tel. No.	Marital Status: □single □married □widowed □divorced		
D.O.B.	Age:	Sex: □male □female	
Spouse's Name:	Children's Names:		

Notes: **widow**「未亡人」 **divorce**「離婚」 **spouse**「配偶者」 **D.O.B**（date of birth）「生年月日」

3. PATIENT-NURSE RELATIONSHIPS

[Step 2]

どちらかがNurseになり、相手（患者役）にDialogue Practiceで練習した質問をして空欄をうめましょう。役割をかえて同様にしてみましょう。

Surname:		Given Name:	
Address:			
Tel. No.	Marital Status: □single □married □widowed □divorced		
D.O.B.	Age:	Sex: □male □female	
Spouse's Name:	Children's Names:		

✚ Dialogue Practice B

患者さんに ①その日の状態 ②ほしいもの ③きらいなもの などをきく練習です。

1．下記のDialogueを読んで、空所を補ってみましょう。
2．CDを聴いて確かめましょう。
3．パートナーと練習してみましょう。

Dialogue　　（A: Nurse　B: Mrs. Patella）

Mrs.Patella 入院2日目の朝に…。

A: How are you feeling today, Mrs. Patella?

B: *Oh, not too bad. But I have a slight headache.* ············①

A: Oh dear. I'll give you something for it. Is there anything else you want?

B: Um. _____ *a newspaper, please*? ········②

A: Sure. By the way, we have lunch at about 11.50. Is there any food which you don't like?

B: _____ *and er, I don't like, er,* _____. ············③

A: Just broccoli and pork sausages?

B: Yes.

✚ Pair Work

[Step 1]

自分が入院していると仮定して、①その日の状態 ②ほしいもの をあらわしているものを囲んでみましょう。また、③嫌いな食べ物はどれですか。印をつけましょう。

① You are feeling   good ／ fine ／ very bad (ill).
    You are   too hot ／ cold ／ hungry ／ very itchy.
    Your leg ／ arm ／ stomach ／   is hurting.

② You want   water ／ coffee ／ tissues ／ a quieter place
                   to watch TV ／ to read a book
                   to use a telephone.

③ ☐ ginger   ☐ grapefruit   ☐ liver   ☐ natto
    ☐ onions   ☐ peppers   ☐ pickles   ☐ pork
    ☐ prunes   ☐ raisins   ☐ raw fish   ☐ watermelon

Notes: **stomach**「胃」(p.90の図参照)   **itchy**「かゆい」

[Step 2]

パートナーと、NurseとPatient間の会話をしてみましょう。Patientになった人はstep 1の情報をDialogue Practice B のイタリックの部分に入れ替えて、Nurseの質問に答えてみましょう。役割をかえてしてみましょう。

Chapter 4

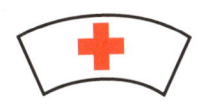

COMMUNICATION WITH A PATIENT

1. Good Communication with a Patient Is Important

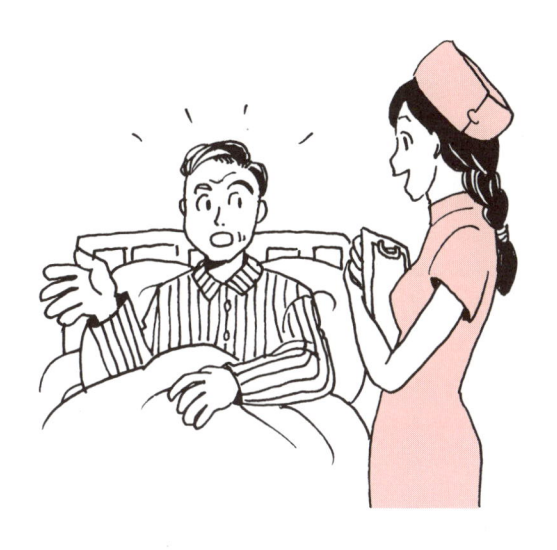

Communication skills are some of the most powerful tools that nurses use in working with patients. It is difficult to really *hear* what the patient is saying to the nurse, and to have the patient really *hear* what the nurse is saying to him or her. It requires time, practice, and desire for the nurse to learn these skills.

Listening skills are often the most difficult for nurses to learn. It is often easier to ask patients lots of questions than to listen quietly to what they have to say. True listening requires that the nurse sit close to the patient, look at the patient, and show interest in what the patient is saying. The best listeners say very little but are able to get the patient to talk. Echoing what the patient says, saying "hmm", and nodding your head are all helpful in getting the patient to talk. Watch patients carefully while they speak. What does their "body language" tell you?

15 In questioning the patient, the nurse should ask open-ended questions that will encourage the patient to talk. Questions that make clear or summarize what the patient has said are very useful for collecting information. Avoid asking questions that require only a "yes" or "no" answer.

Notes: コミュニケーション技術は、看護師の最も強力な道具の１つ。
have the patient really *hear* 「患者に本当に聞いてもらう」have＋人＋原形動詞で haveは使役（させる、してもらう）。 **It requires ... for the nurse to ～** 「看護師が～するには…を要する」Itは仮主語。 **desire** 「意欲」 **requires that the nurse ...** 「看護師が…することを要する」require（要求する）に続くthat節では動詞の原形が使われる点にも注意。 **The best listeners** 「聞くのが最も上手な人、聞き方の名人」 **get the patient to talk** 「患者に話させる」３行目のhaveと同様getも使役動詞。ただし、getはto の付いた不定詞（to talk）を従える。 **open-ended questions** 「自由に回答できる形式の質問」選択肢から選ぶのでなく。

✚ Vocabulary

Fill in each blank with one word from the list below. Use each of them only once.

[communication skills practice body language
information]

1. The nurse tried to gain detailed (　　　) about the patient.
2. Patients use (　　　) to show their feelings to nurses.
3. The nurse must have good (　　　) with the patient.
4. It takes a lot of (　　　) to be really good at questioning the patient.
5. The nurse has to learn the (　　　) of listening to the patient.

4. COMMUNICATION WITH A PATIENT

✚ Questions & Answers

> 1. 2. Choose the best answer.
> 3. 4. Answer in English.
> 5. Make your own question.

1. What is the most difficult communication skill?
   a. asking   b. listening   c. speaking

2. What do the best listeners do?
   a. They get the patient to talk.
   b. They talk a lot with patients.
   c. They stop the patient from talking.

3. How can you get the patient to talk?
   _____
   _____

4. How should the nurse question the patient?
   _____
   _____

5. Your question _____
   _____
   Answer _____

✚ Grammar & Usage

> Fill in each blank with one word from the list below. Use each of them only once.

[make   cause   get   encourage   let]

1. Nurses often (   ) patients to give up smoking.
2. Whenever I see the nurse, she tries to (   ) me laugh.
3. The nurse tried to (   ) the patient to talk about herself.
4. Heavy drinking can (   ) people to drive carelessly.
5. Please (   ) me know what happens.

2. Thank You for Talking to Me

Dialogue A ⟨A: Nurse   B: Patient⟩

手術前で不安な様子の患者に…。

A: You look very sad.

B: Yes, nurse. I'm frightened.

A: What are you concerned about?

B: I'm afraid I won't live through my surgery. I'm scared of dying.

A: You think you will die?

B: I'm afraid I'll go to sleep and never wake up.

A: Do you know why you're so worried about this?

B: I'm not sure. Maybe it's because my mother died when she had surgery.

A: So you are worried that the same thing will happen to you?

B: Yes. I guess so. Can you do something to help me relax?

A: The doctor asked me to give you an injection to help you relax. You'll remember going into the operating room. Then you'll see me when you wake up.

B: Thank you for talking to me. I feel better now.

Notes: **be frightened**「こわがる、こわい」   **be concerned about**〜「〜について心配する」
be worried about〜「〜を心配する」   **surgery**「手術」   **operating room**「手術室」

Dialogue B ⟨A: Nurse Knight   B: Little Girl⟩

定期健康診断をうけにきた少女に…。

A: Hi Suzy. Wow! You're getting big. Let's see how heavy you are! Just stand on this scale here.	要請、命令
B: What does it say?	質問
A: 18. 18 kilograms. You are growing! Can I see your teeth? Show me your teeth…. Ooh!!! Some teeth came out.	答え、要請、命令
B: I got some money from the Tooth Fairy.	自慢
A: Great! But you look worried about something.	間接的問いかけ
B: Do I have to get a shot today?	質問
A: No, Suzy. That's all for today's check-up. You can go home now.	答え、終わる
B: Bye bye.	

4. COMMUNICATION WITH A PATIENT

✚ True or False (Dialogue A)

> Listen and write what you hear. Then circle T (true) or F (false).

1. _____ T / F
2. _____ T / F
3. _____ T / F
4. _____ T / F
5. _____ T / F

✚ Dialogue Practice (Dialogue B)

> **1.** Substitute the words shown below.

▶ sentence: Let's see **how heavy you are!**
 1. tall → _____
 2. your blood pressure → _____
 3. your temperature → _____
 4. touchy, it → _____

▶ sentence: **Can I see your teeth?**
 1. May → _____
 2. Could → _____
 3. hands → _____
 4. fingers → _____

> **2.** Practice the dialogue.

✚ Vocabulary (Dialogues A and B)

> Choose the word that means the same as the expression on the right, as it is used in the text.

1. frightened   ( )   a. place where surgery is performed
2. concerned   ( )   b. injection
3. operating room ( )   c. physical examination
4. shot   ( )   d. scared
5. check-up   ( )   e. worried

3. LET'S TALK: Listening to and Sympathizing with the Patient

🎧 34 ✚ Vocabulary

各々の絵を記述している英語はどれでしょう。（番号で答えましょう）

- to have an accident ( )
- to be burnt down ( )
- to be bitten by a snake ( )
- to be late / to be in a hurry ( )
- to be sad ( )
- to fall off a horse ( )
- to have an operation ( )
- to die ( )

4. COMMUNICATION WITH A PATIENT

✚ Listen to the story

1. CDのstoryをよく聴きましょう。前ページの1～10のどの絵に関連があるか、その番号を○でかこみましょう。

2. CDのstoryについて質問に答えましょう。

    1. What happened?　　　　_____

    2. When did it happen?　　_____

    3. Where did it happen?　　_____

    4. How did the speaker feel?_____

3. もう一度CDを聴きましょう。（質問の仕方にも注意しましょう）

✚ Listen to your partner's story

1. **Vocabulary**の1～10にならって、11と12の枠にどうして病院に来たかについての絵を自分で描いてみましょう。

2. 1～12の絵のうちの5つか6つを使ってあなたのstoryを創って書いてみましょう。その場合、**Listen to the story**の4つの質問（順序は問いません）に答えられるようにしましょう。

3. パートナーにあなたの話をしましょう。（できるだけ書いたものを見ないで話すようにしましょう。）

4．パートナーはよく相手の話を聴きましょう。聴きながら次の英語を使って
相手に対する共感を伝えてみましょう。

That's sad.
That's a shame.
It's a pity.
I'm sorry to hear that.

5．パートナーの話について質問に答えましょう。

1. What happened? _____
   _____

2. When did it happen? _____
   _____

3. Where did it happen? _____
   _____

4. How did the speaker feel? _____
   _____

6．役割をかえて同様にしてみましょう。

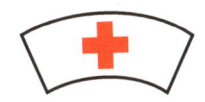

Chapter 5
INTERCULTURAL COMMUNICATION WITH A PATIENT

1. How Can Culture Cause Problems?

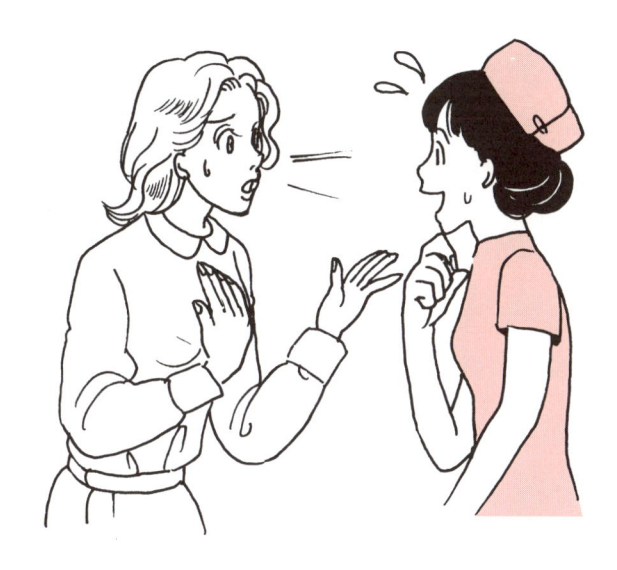

Nursing is closely involved with some of the most important events of a person's life: when a child is born, when someone becomes critically ill, or when someone is dying. These events are usually filled with emotion, meaning, or tradition. However, the meaning of these events to the patient may be very different depending upon the cultural beliefs of the patient.

Many nurses feel awkward and uncomfortable when they talk with someone from another culture. The nurse should be able to be helpful to any patient going through a crisis. This requires the nurse to recognize and value how people are different. Nurses cannot accurately tell whether patients have a problem or how to help them without understanding the cultural meaning of the event for the patients.

15 　　Language is often a barrier to understanding. Sometimes patients speak different languages, or they may use the same words, but the meaning is different.

　　In talking to patients, the nurse should ask if they have any special beliefs or things they do when they are ill. Ask them about what they like to eat or unusual medicines they might take. Inquire
20 about whether they have a spiritual leader who should be called. See if there is anything special they would like you to do for them, or anything you should avoid.

Notes: 看護は出産のような人の生涯の非常に重要な部分と密接に関係している。 **is closely involved with…**「…と密接に関係している」　**becomes critically ill**「危篤になる」　**event(s)**「重大事」　**depending upon the cultural beliefs**「文化的信条によって」　**feel awkward and uncomfortable**「気まずく落ち着かない感じがする」　**going through…**「…を通り抜けつつある、…を乗り切ろうとしている」　**the cultural meaning of the event for the patients**「その患者にとってのその重大事の文化的意味」　**barrier**「障害」　**unusual medicines**「風変わりな薬」　**spiritual leader**「精神的な指導者、魂の指導者」

38 ✚ Vocabulary

Match the similar expressions.

1. critical　　（　）
2. traditions　（　）
3. emotions　 （　）
4. crisis　　　（　）
5. accurate　 （　）

a. beliefs and customs passed down from the past to the present
b. strong feelings such as love, hate, desire or fear
c. serious situation which needs attention quickly
d. careful and exact
e. very serious and dangerous

5. INTERCULTURAL COMMUNICATION WITH A PATIENT

✚ Questions & Answers

> 1. 2. Choose the best answer.
> 3. 4. Answer in English.
> 5. Make your own question.

1. How is the nurse likely to feel toward the patient from another culture?
   a. curious   b. ill at ease   c. relaxed

2. What should the nurse know when caring for the patient from another culture?
   a. where the patient comes from
   b. how people are different
   c. what language the patient speaks

3. What should the nurse understand to help the patient from another culture with his problem?
   _____

4. What should the nurse ask patients from other cultures?
   _____
   _____

5. Your question _____
   _____
   Answer _____

✚ Grammar & Usage

> Fill in each blank with one word from the list below. Use each of them only once.

[how   if   that   what   whether]

1. Yumi has learnt (   ) the nurse must make a holistic assessment of the patient.
2. The nurse asked Jed (   ) he wanted to read a book.
3. The nurse didn't understand (   ) Mr. Kim told her.
4. It is doubtful (   ) Julie will recover or not.
5. The nurse had no idea (   ) the patient from India felt about a bed-bath.

2. Something Special for Me

Dialogue A ⟨A: Nurse　B: Woman⟩

American Indianの女性が出産を終えて…。

A: You worked very hard having that baby. Now you know why they call it labor. Maybe you'd like some cold orange juice.

B: Could I have a glass of warm tea?

A: Sure. Is there some reason you don't want orange juice?

B: Well, yes. You may laugh at me, but my mother taught me that I should not drink anything cold or eat any meat while I'm still bleeding.

A: I didn't realize that was one of your beliefs. Of course I'll get you some warm tea. Is there anything else you'd like?

B: I'd very much like to be alone. This is a sacred time for me. Now that I have a baby, I've a lot to think about.

A: Of course. I'll put a sign on your door so others won't disturb you. That way you can have some privacy.

B: Thanks.

Notes:　**labor**「分娩、陣痛、(骨折り)」　**bleed**「出血する」 *cf.* blood「血」

Dialogue B ⟨A: Mother　B: Nurse⟩

バイクに乗った少年が車にはねられ病院に運び込まれた。彼の母親が病院に駆けつけて…。

A: Nurse, can you tell me how Jeremy is?	質問
B: I'm afraid he cut his leg pretty badly. He has lost a lot of blood, but he should be OK.	答え
A: Lost a lot of blood?	繰り返し
B: Yes. We're going to give him a transfusion.	予定提言
A: No. You can't do that. We are not allowed.	反対
B: Eh!! W' W' what do you mean?	問いかけ
A: Our religion doesn't allow it. Blood transfusion.	説明

Notes:　**transfusion**「輸血」　**religion**「宗教」

5. INTERCULTURAL COMMUNICATION WITH A PATIENT

✚ True or False (Dialogue A)

Listen and write what you hear. Then circle T (true) or F (false).

1. _____ T / F
2. _____ T / F
3. _____ T / F
4. _____ T / F
5. _____ T / F

✚ Dialogue Practice (Dialogue B)

1. Substitute the words shown below.

▶ sentence: I am afraid **he badly cut his leg.**
 1. she → _____
 2. hand → _____
 3. severely burn → _____
 4. seriously injure → _____

▶ sentence: **We're going to give him a transfusion.**
 1. The doctor → _____
 2. her → _____
 3. injection → _____
 4. X-ray treatment → _____

2. Practice the dialogue.

✚ Vocabulary (Dialogues A and B)

Fill in each blank with one word from the list below. Use each of them only once.

[labor   belief   privacy   transfusion   religion]

1. The patient did not express his (   ) in Christianity.
2. The patient receives a blood (   ) every two weeks.
3. My (   ) forbids me to eat pork.
4. The patient did not want anybody to disturb her (   ).
5. The mother had a difficult (   ), but forgot it when she saw her baby.

3. LET'S TALK: Avoiding and Solving Difficulties

✚ What Is the Problem?

1. 次の絵の中の患者さんは文化の違いから生じる問題で困っています。何が問題なのか考えてみましょう。問題は一つとは限りません。例の絵の患者さんは：

   The patient seems unhappy.
   The bed's too small.
   Also, the bed's too hard.
   The patient's cold.

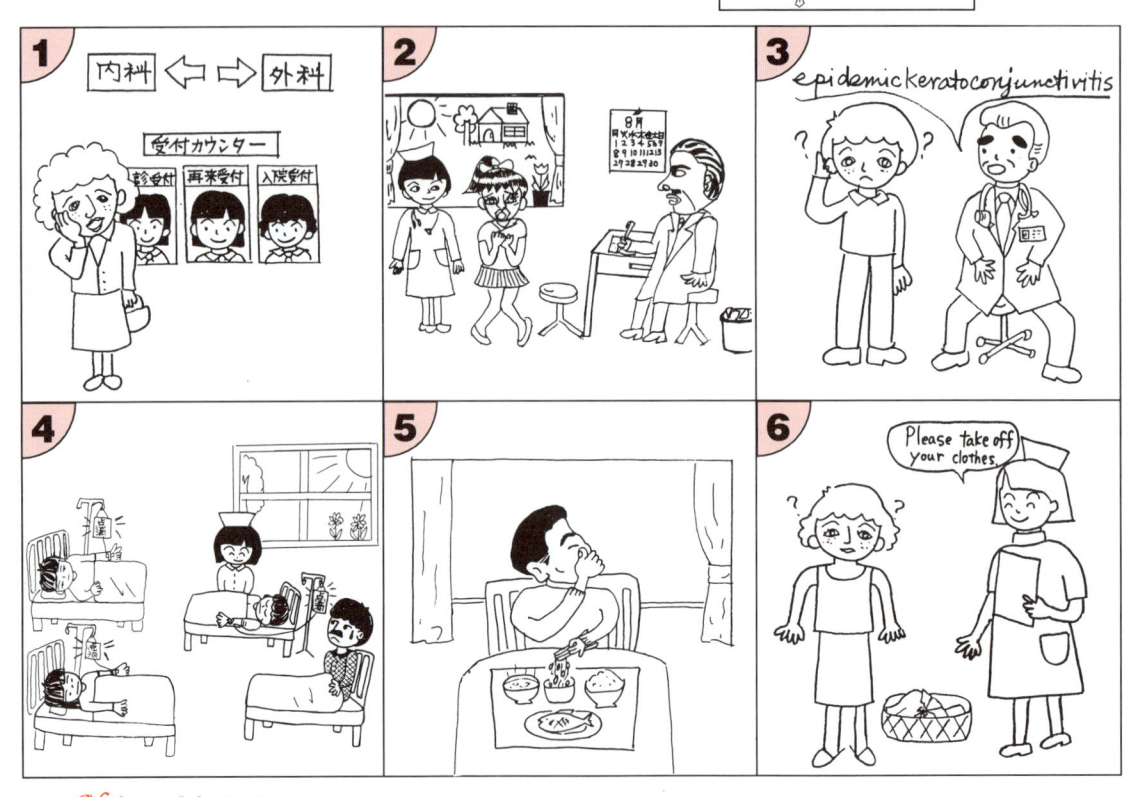

Notes: drip「点滴」

5. INTERCULTURAL COMMUNICATION WITH A PATIENT

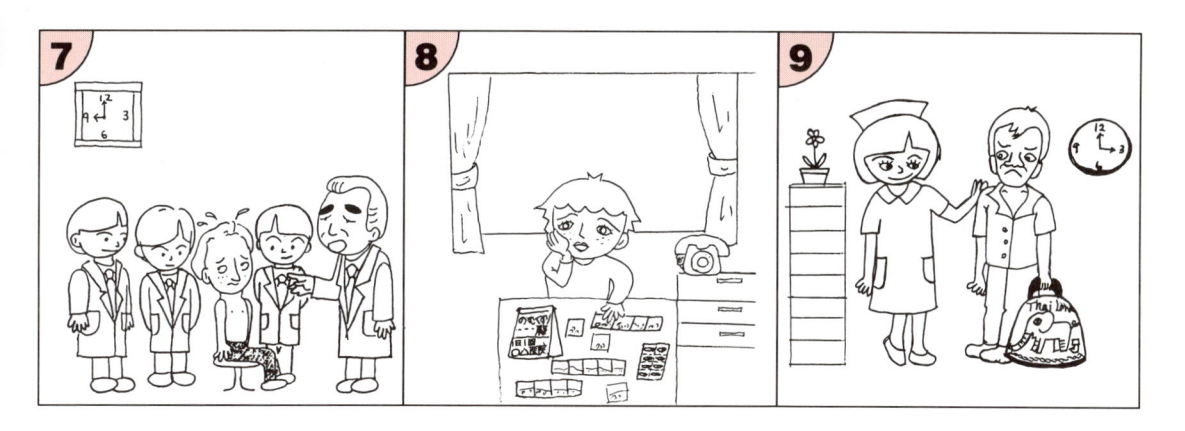

43 2. 各々の絵の患者さんの困っていることについてパートナーと例にならって dialogue してみましょう。

[例]

A: What do you think is the problem?	質問
B: *I think* that the bed's too short for the patient.	答え
A: *Yes, I agree.* The patient's very tall.	同意

44 3. できればさらに次のように dialogue を発展させてみましょう。

[例]

A: What do you think is the problem?	質問
B: *I think* that the bed's too short for the patient.	答え（言明）
A: *Yes, I agree.* The patient's very tall. I think that *maybe* the bed is also too hard.	同意
B: *I'm not sure I agree.* But I think that the patient feels cold.	疑問、新たな言明
A: *Yes, perhaps* he has a fever.	同意、支持言明

4．例にならって患者さんのためにしてあげられることを話し合ってみましょう。

[例]

A: I think *we should* give him a larger bed.	示唆
B: Ah, *but* maybe all the beds are too small.	反論
A: *Then* perhaps hospitals should all have one or two very large beds. Then they *can* give the large beds to very tall people.	別の示唆
B: *That's a good idea.*	同意

5．ペア毎に一つの絵を選び、例にならってNurseと患者間の会話をつくってみましょう。

[例]　（A: Nurse　B: Mr. Sand）

A: *How are you,* Mr. Sand?	あいさつ
B: Oh! My back aches* because the bed's too small.	不平
A: Oh dear! *I'm sorry,* Mr. Sand. None of the beds in our department are large enough. *We're going to* bring you another bed from another department right away.	謝り（共感） 問題の説明 解決の説明
B: Great! That'll be nice.	感謝
A: *Anything else I can do*?	援助の申し出
B: *Could you* give me another blanket? I'm cold.	要請
A: *Certainly.*	引き受け

＊ache [éik]「ずきずき痛む」

6．パートナーと練習してみましょう。

7．皆の前で発表してみましょう。

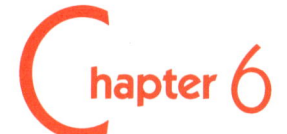

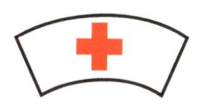

Chapter 6
DOCTOR-NURSE RELATIONSHIP

1. Nurses Work Closely with Doctors

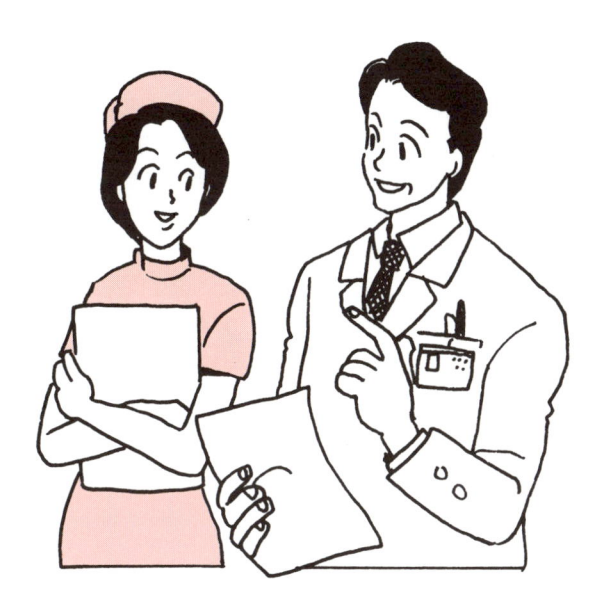

In most cultures, nursing is done by women. Some nursing duties are similar to the work women do for their families. As more scientific knowledge is learned, many nursing tasks become less like work in the home. The work is very important and requires special education and critical thinking.

The majority of nursing care is provided in hospitals. Basic nursing care is given every day to keep patients clean and safe. As doctors spend more of their time in surgery or in their offices, they rely on the nurses to care for the patients. Special procedures, tests, and medications are ordered by physicians. Nurses work closely with physicians to see that the orders are carried out. Nurses not

only help feed and bathe the patients but also report to the physicians about what they observe. They tell the doctor how the patients respond to the treatments and medicines. They learn about
15 the patients' concerns and worries that delay their recovery. They write what they see in the chart. The physicians depend on the information in the chart to help them plan what to do next. The knowledge and skills of both groups help the patient get well.

Notes: ほとんどの文化圏において看護は女性によってなされる。なぜ？
As more scientific knowledge is learned「科学的知識が増えるにつれて」 **critical thinking**「批判的思考」 **nursing care**「看護」 **office**「診察室」 **rely on ... to ~**「…が～するのをあてにする」 **procedure(s)**「処置」 **medication(s)**「薬剤」可算語のとき medicine と同じ。 **work closely with ... to see that ~**「～されるように取り計らうために…と緊密に連絡をとり合う、…と緊密に連絡をとり合って確実に～されるようにする」 **concerns and worries**「懸念や心配」 **in the chart**「カルテに」この句はすぐ前の see でなく離れた write を修飾する。 **depend on ... to ~** *cf.* Chap.2

48 ✚ Vocabulary

Match the similar expressions.

1. duty   (　)   a. paper with information written
2. treatment   (　)   about a patient
3. chart   (　)   b. getting well
4. recovery   (　)   c. what one must do because of
5. medication (　)   one's job
                       d. drug
                       e. act of curing by medical means

6. DOCTOR-NURSE RELATIONSHIP

✚ Questions & Answers

> 1. 2. Choose the best answer.
> 3. 4. Answer in English.
> 5. Make your own question.

1. Who mainly cares for patients in hospitals?
   a. doctors   b. family   c. nurses

2. Who mainly orders procedures, tests and medications?
   a. doctors   b. family   c. nurses

3. What jobs do nurses do for patients?
   _____
   _____

4. What do nurses tell doctors about patients?
   _____
   _____

5. Your question _____
   Answer _____

✚ Grammar & Usage

> Fill in each blank with one pair of words from the list below. Use each of them only once.

[belong to   care for   carry out   depend on   respond to]

1. Patients will never forget nurses who (   ) them tenderly in their stay in the hospital.
2. The disease does not (   ) the new drug.
3. She always tried to (   ) a plan to make patients comfortable.
4. Doctors (   ) nurses in gaining information about patients.
5. Today an increasing number of physicians (   ) large hospitals.

2. That's Important Information

Dialogue A ⟨A: Doctor   B: Nurse⟩

退院する Mrs. White の今後のことを気遣って…。

A: Mrs. White is ready to go home now. Her lungs are clear and she has no wheezing.

B: Yes, she seems much better.

A: I want to send some asthma medicine home with her. Please explain to her how to use the medicine before she leaves.

B: The family seems very concerned about taking care of her when she gets home. Perhaps we ought to ask a community health nurse to stop by the home and work with the family.

A: That's a good idea. A community health nurse can help teach the patient some breathing exercises for her asthma and make sure that her lungs are clear.

B: I'll call a community health nurse and we'll have a family conference before the patient is discharged.

A: That's an excellent idea.

Notes   **asthma**「喘息」   **community health nurse**「地域保健婦」   **discharge**「退院させる」

Dialogue B ⟨A: Nurse   B: Doctor⟩

肺に感染のある Mr. Black について…。

A: Mr. Black said that he's allergic to penicillin.	情報を提供
B: Oh dear!	理解
A: It gives him a rash and makes him itch.	さらに情報を提供
B: OK. Let's try erythromycin.	代わりの指示
A: How much should I give him?	指示をあおぐ
B: Umm. By drip 800mg. But first make sure that he's not allergic to it.	答え

Notes   **allergic**「アレルギー体質の」   **rash**「発疹」   **itch**「かゆい」   **erythromycin**「エリスロマイシン（感染症の治療に用いる抗生物質）」   **drip**「点滴」

6. DOCTOR-NURSE RELATIONSHIP

➕ True or False (Dialogue A)

> Listen and write what you hear. Then circle T (true) or F (false).

1. _____ T / F
2. _____ T / F
3. _____ T / F
4. _____ T / F
5. _____ T / F

➕ Dialogue Practice (Dialogue B)

> **1.** Substitute the words shown below.

▶ sentence: **Mr. Black said that he's allergic to penicillin.**
  1. Mrs. White → _____
  2. milk → _____
  3. had a severe headache → _____

▶ sentence: **How much should I give him?**
  1. her → _____
  2. many tablets → _____
  3. What → _____

> **2.** Practice the dialogue.

➕ Vocabulary (Dialogues A and B)

> Choose the word that means the same as the expression on the right, as it is used in the text.

1. asthma   ( )   a. hypersensitivity to something
2. discharge ( )   b. condition which makes breathing very difficult at times
3. allergy   ( )   c. red spots on the face or body caused by illness
4. rash   ( )   d. feel a soreness which one wants to scratch
5. itch   ( )   e. allow to leave the hospital

3. LET'S TALK: The Nurse Seeks Advice from the Doctor

➕ Vocabulary (Pair Work)

1. 各語群（7語）のspellingをパートナーに読みあげてもらって書きとりましょう。
2. 各語の意味を調べましょう。CDを聞いて発音しましょう。

| suppository / catheter / drip / elderly / dehydrated / wrinkled / appetite | vital signs / pulse / respiration / urine / paralyzed / bed-ridden / pneumonia |

➕ Dialogue Practice

1. CDを聴いて空所をうめましょう。1語とは限りません。
2. 右側に例にならって会話の構成を書いてみましょう。
3. パートナーと練習しましょう。

NurseがDoctorに電話で患者の治療について助言を求めて…。〈A: Nurse　B: Doctor〉

A: Hello, Doctor Watson, I'm Nurse Temple at Saint Mary's Home for the Elderly.　　例：あいさつ、自己紹介
B: Good morning, Nurse Temple. What can I do for you?　　_____
A: I think that one of our _____ dehydrated.　　_____
B: Her vital signs?　　_____
A: _____ 95. Temp 37.7. Respiration 24.　　_____
B: And her intake and _____?　　_____

B: Yes, it seems like she is _____.　　_____
A: Shall I give her a drip?　　_____
B: Yes. Solita T3.　　_____
A: _____ much?　　_____
B: 500cc. One _____.　　_____
A: 12 hours?　　_____

➕ Role Play (Pair Work): Working in a Home for the Elderly

1. 高齢者ホームの患者さんについてNurseがDoctorに電話する会話です。NurseとDoctorのどちらになるかを決め、自分の役割の **Card** をよく読みましょう。
2. 指示に従い、患者さんの状態に沿った内容の会話を自由にしてみましょう。

6. DOCTOR-NURSE RELATIONSHIP

【Nurse Card】

> ◆ 設定 ◆
>
> あなたはManchesterにあるBartlet's Home for the Elderly（高齢者ホーム）に働くNurseです。
>
> ある患者さんが食欲が落ち、飲み物も殆ど飲まなくなりました。皮膚が以前よりずっと乾燥（dry）し、しわがよった（wrinkled）状態になりました。今までの経験上、多分脱水状態（dehydrated）だと思われます。あなたは確認と指示を得るため医師に電話することにしました。

1. まずPatient's Recordを読みましょう。
2. Nurse Notesを読んで医師に何を聞きたいかよく考えておきましょう。
3. Dialogue Practice (p.52) を参考にして会話を始めましょう。
4. Doctorは結論を言う前にあなたに患者さんについていろいろ聞くでしょう。Patient's Recordをみてできるだけ情報を伝えましょう。
5. Doctorの指示を聞き取ってメモしましょう。

【Nurse Notes】

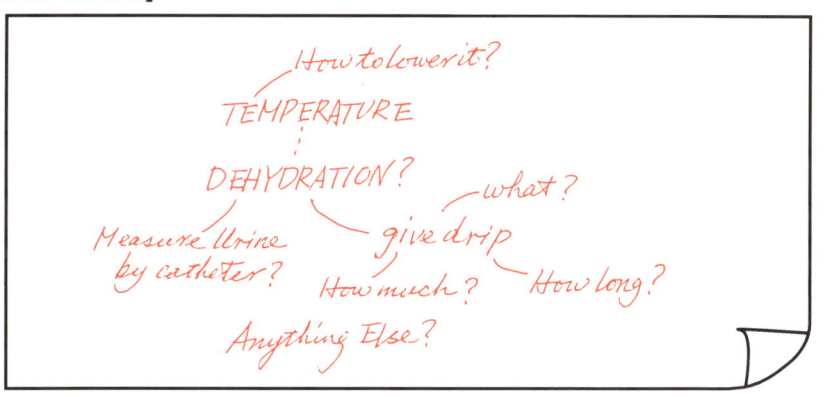

```
              How to lower it?
              TEMPERATURE
                   ⋮
              DEHYDRATION?         what?
                                    ╲
Measure Urine          give drip
by catheter?      How much?    How long?
              Anything Else?
```

Patient's Record

SURNAME: Liver	FIRST NAME: Dolly	AGE: 92
BACKGROUND INFORMATION	Bedridden (stroke 5 years ago) Paralyzed (left half of body)	
MEDICATION: None		
TEMPERATURE: 37.8℃	PULSE: 100	RESPIRATION: 24
PRESENT CONDITION:	loss of appetite & drinks little unusually dry wrinkled skin difficulty in breathing only small amount of urine mood is not good	

【Doctor Card】

> ◆ 設定 ◆
>
> あなたはManchesterのある病院に勤務する老人病科の医師です。あなたの患者さんの多くは外来患者ですが、他の病院に入院している人もいます。Nurseから電話があります。まず自己紹介した後、治療についてあなたの助言を聞きます。

1. まずTreatment Card（治療カード）をよく読んでおきましょう。
2. Dialogue Practice（p.52）を参考にして会話をしましょう。
3. 助言する前に患者さんについて情報が必要です。現在の状態では何が重要な情報か考え、重要なものからNurseに聞きだしてPatient's Recordに書き込みましょう。
4. Nurseから得た情報では患者は脱水症状(dehydrated)を呈しています。Nurseにそのことを伝えましょう。
5. どうすればよいかについてのNurseの質問にTreatment Cardの情報を使って答えましょう。

Patient's Record

SURNAME:	FIRST NAME:	AGE:
CURRENT MEDICATION*		
TEMPERATURE:	PULSE:	RESPIRATION:
PRESENT CONDITION:		

* current medication　患者の現在の投薬

Treatment Card

Illness: Most likely dehydration but also may be pneumonia.

For fever: If T above 38℃ then Voltaren suppository.

If T below 38℃ then cool with ice pack.

Drip: Solita T3 (500 cc)　two bottles　24 hrs

Take for chest X-ray—need to check whether it is pneumonia.

Measure amount of urine—need to check intake and output (don't use catheter).

Food: Light meals OK

Chapter 7

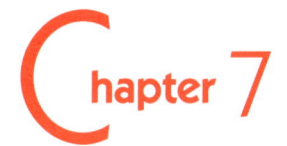

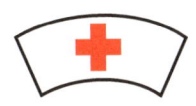

RELATED PROFESSIONALS

1. Nurses Work with Related Professionals

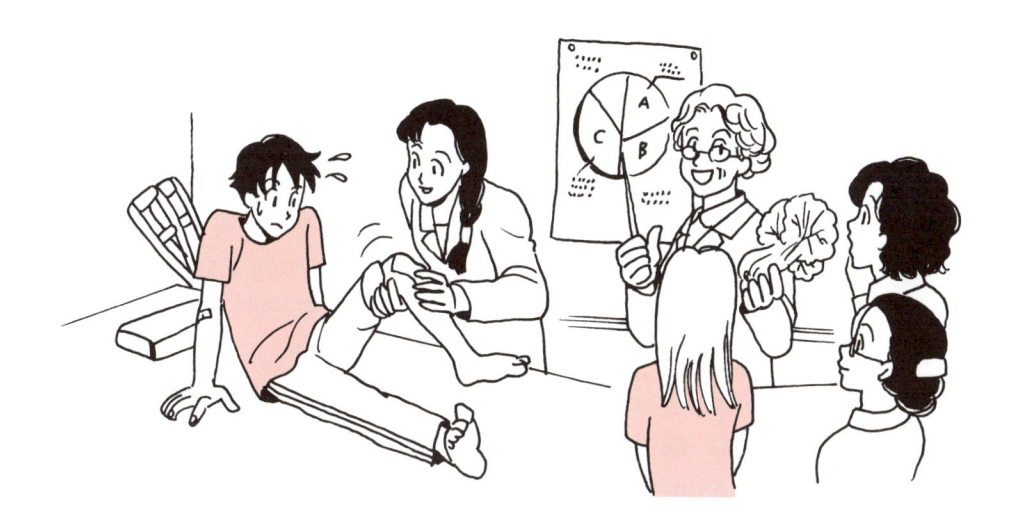

The first nurses did everything needed to care for the patient. Besides cooking, cleaning and bathing, they gave medicine, started oxygen, did dressings and other procedures. Over time, other health care providers performed many of these duties.

As more was known about nutrition, dietitians directed the cooking and serving of food. As technology developed, radiologists, physical therapists, and other specialties grew to assist in the diagnosis and treatment of patients. Pharmacists began mixing and delivering all the drugs. Physical therapists helped the patients re-train their muscles and nerves. Respiratory therapists took over the equipment that eased breathing problems. Discharge nurses

worked with social workers to help patients obtain the community resources they needed when they went home.   The increasing number of people working together created a need for good leaders:
15 administrators, nursing and medical directors, and supervisors.

　　　　Hospitals or clinics require many individuals to meet the needs of patients.   They all perform essential work as part of the health care team.

Notes: 最初に看護師になった人々は、患者さんを看護するために必要なことは何でもやった。
started oxygen ＜ start oxygen「酸素をスタートさせる」酸素マスクなどの装置で酸素を投与するために栓をひねるなどすること。   **did dressings** ＜ do dressings「包帯を巻く」   **nutrition**「栄養」   **dietitians directed ...**「栄養士が…を監督するようになった」   **develop**「発達する」   **radiologist(s)**「放射線専門家」   **physical therapist(s)**「理学療法士」   **specialties** ＜ specialty「専門」 **... grew to assist ～**「…が登場して～ を助けるようになった」   **diagnosis**「診断」   **delivering** ＜ deliver「手渡す」   **re-train ...**「…を再訓練する」   **respiratory therapist(s)**「呼吸療法士」重症な呼吸障害をもつ患者の管理・治療を助ける。   **took over ...** ＜ take over ...「…を引き受ける」   **discharge nurse(s)**「退院看護師」   **administrators**「管理運営にあたる人々」   **nursing and medical directors and supervisors**「看護部長・診療部長や婦長・医長」   **part of the health care team**「医療チームの一員」

✚ Vocabulary

Match the similar expressions.

1. dressing　　（　）
2. respiration　（　）
3. diagnosis　　（　）
4. dietitian　　（　）
5. pharmacist　 （　）

a. person trained in the science of food and drink
b. person skilled in the making of medicines
c. covering on a wound
d. breathing
e. identifying a disease from its signs and symptoms

7. RELATED PROFESSIONALS

✚ Questions & Answers

> 1. 2. Choose the best answer.
> 3. 4. Answer in English.
> 5. Make your own question.

1. What didn't the nurses do for the patient?
   a. clean wounds   b. perform surgery
   c. give food

2. Which professional is most concerned with the diagnosis of the patient?
   a. the dietitian   b. the radiologist
   c. the discharge nurse

3. What do pharmacists do?
   _____
   _____

4. What do respiratory therapists do?
   _____
   _____

5. Your question _____
   _____
   Answer _____

✚ Grammar & Usage

> Write the correct form of the verb.

1. The medicine (　　　　) to the patient had a powerful effect. [give]
2. The patient (　　　　) little about his disease when he was hospitalized. [know]
3. Dietitians, (　　　　) care of patients' nutrition, direct the cooking and serving of food. [take]
4. The radiologist helps (　　　　) the patient's cancer. [treat]
5. Besides (　　　　) carefully to patients, the nurse should also observe their body language. [listen]

57 ▶▶▶

2. Work as Part of the Health Care Team

Dialogue A 〈A: Dietitian B: Patient〉

physical therapistと歩行訓練の話を終えて…。

A: Hello, Mr. Wilson. Remember me?

B: I'm sorry, I don't. There are so many people in the hospital I get mixed up.

A: I'm Ms. Tanaka, the dietitian who stopped by yesterday to discuss the new diet the resident ordered for you.

B: Oh, Yes! Now, I remember.

A: How was lunch today?

B: Well, I haven't had a chance to eat yet. I was in physical therapy when the tray came.

A: Are you just going to practice walking with your crutches?

B: I guess it will depend upon how short of breath I am.

A: Well, it sounds like we need to schedule activities better so you don't miss your meals.

B: Thanks. That would help.

Notes: **dietitian**「栄養士」 **resident**「レジデント（専門医になるための研修をうけている医師）」 **physical therapy**「理学療法」 **crutch**「松葉杖」

Dialogue B 〈A: Student Nurse B: Supervisor〉

Mrs. Grant宅を訪問したことを報告して…。　(Mr. Green: Social Worker Ms. Peck: Dietitian)

A: Mrs. Grant's heartbeat was irregular. So I reported it to the physician.	報告
B: Hmm.	応答（うなずき）
A: Later in the week she complained of nausea, blurred vision and dizziness to Mr. Green.	さらに報告
B: It sounds like she's become very ill.	応答（感想）
A: She has! Later on, Ms. Peck found her lying on the floor. She was admitted to the hospital. Blood tests showed that she had high levels of digitalis.	さらに報告
B: Ah…. That explains the irregular heartbeat then.	応答（了解）

Notes: **heartbeat**「心拍（動）」 **blurred vision**「かすみ目」 **dizziness**「めまい」 **admit**「入院させる」 **digitalis**「ジギタリス（強心薬）」

7. RELATED PROFESSIONALS

🞤 True or False (Dialogue A) [CD 58]

Listen and write what you hear. Then circle T (true) or F (false).

1. _____ T / F
2. _____ T / F
3. _____ T / F
4. _____ T / F
5. _____ T / F

🞤 Dialogue Practice (Dialogue B)

1. Substitute the words shown below or follow the instructions.

▶ sentence: **She complained of nausea.**
   1. blurred vision → _____
   2. dizziness → _____
   3. lower back pain → _____
   4. 疑問文 → _____

▶ sentence: **Blood tests showed that she had high levels of digitalis.**
   1. sugar → _____
   2. cholesterol → _____
   3. low levels of iron → _____
   4. 現在形 → _____

2. Practice the dialogue.

🞤 Vocabulary (Dialogues A and B) [CD 60]

Choose the word that means the same as the expression on the right, as it is used in the text.

1. resident   (   )
2. therapy   (   )
3. crutch   (   )
4. vision   (   )
5. dizziness (   )

a. stick for supporting a person with difficulty in walking
b. having a feeling that things are going round and round
c. sight
d. specialist in training
e. treatment of illness

3. LET'S TALK: Consulting a Specialist

✚ Vocabulary

1. 医学用語はギリシャ語、ラテン語を起源としています。ギリシャ、ラテン語と英語を比較しましょう。

Greek or Latin	English
-atrician	person who studies
-ologist	person who studies
-ology	subject, study
derm-	skin
geri-	old
gyneco-	female
hema-	blood
ophthal-	eye
pedi-	child or foot

61 2. 例を参考にして表を完成しましょう。CDを聴いて発音しましょう。

[例] A doctor who specializes in:
- skin is called a *dermatologist* and works in the *dermatology* department.
- children is called a *pediatrician* and works in the *pediatrics* department.

Department	Specialist (English)	Specialist (Japanese)
dermatology	dermatologist	
geriatrics		
gynecology		
hematology		
ophthalmology		
pediatrics	pediatrician	

7. RELATED PROFESSIONALS

3．表の6つのdepartment（科）とspecialist（専門医）を覚えましょう。
4．例にならってクラスのいろいろな人と質問し合いましょう。

[例] • What do you call a doctor who specializes in *blood*?
• In which department do *hematologists* work?

✚ Telling a Story

1．次のA〜Fのstoryのどれか一つをよく読んで情報を覚え、テキストを見ないで他の人に情報を伝えることができるようにしましょう。
2．他のstoryの情報を聴きあいましょう。5回パートナーをかえてA〜Fすべての情報を得るようにしましょう。

A Jane Kawase is 4 years old. Jane was in the kitchen. She was watching her mother cooking. Jane wanted to look inside a pan. When she took the pan, hot water splashed on her body. This hurt her very much and badly damaged her skin. Jane had to go to the hospital. Which specialist treated her?	**B** Jane's grandfather, Bill Kawase, is very old. He has many problems. For example, he cannot see very well, he cannot hear very well, and he cannot walk. He sits in a wheelchair and the nurses push him. A doctor often examines him. What type of doctor often examines him?
C Jane's brother, Peter Kawase, is 6 years old. Two days ago, his stomach started to hurt. He went to his family doctor. His family doctor sent him to the hospital. Now, Peter's staying in the children's ward. What type of doctor examined his stomach and gave him some medicine?	**D** Jane's father, John Kawase, likes to play tennis. Last week he was playing tennis with his friend. The ball hit Mr. Kawase in the left eye. His eye was damaged. Mr. Kawase went to the hospital. Which type of doctor probably examined Mr. Kawase's eye?
E Jane's mother, Helen Kawase, is a nurse. Since last week she has been very tired every day. She also has a high temperature. Maybe she has caught an infection from a patient. A doctor took a blood sample. What type of doctor examined the blood sample?	**F** Last week, Jane's sister, Kate, went swimming near her house. There, the sea is not clean. Three days ago her period started. It was much more painful than normal. Also the color of the blood was a little strange. She feels very itchy. Maybe she has an infection. Which type of doctor should she visit?

Notes: infection「感染」 period「月経」

3. 次の質問に答えましょう。

1. Jane visited the dermatologist. Why?
   _____
   _____

2. How was Mr. Kawase's eye damaged?
   _____
   _____

3. What type of sample did the doctor take from Jane's mother?
   _____
   _____

4. How did Jane's sister get an infection?
   _____
   _____

5. Why does Jane's grandfather have many problems?
   _____
   _____

6. Which part of Peter's body was hurting?
   _____
   _____

Chapter 8

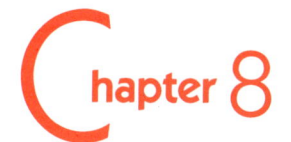

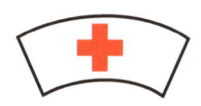

NURSES AND THE HOSPITAL

1. The Work Nurses Do Depends on the Type of Hospital

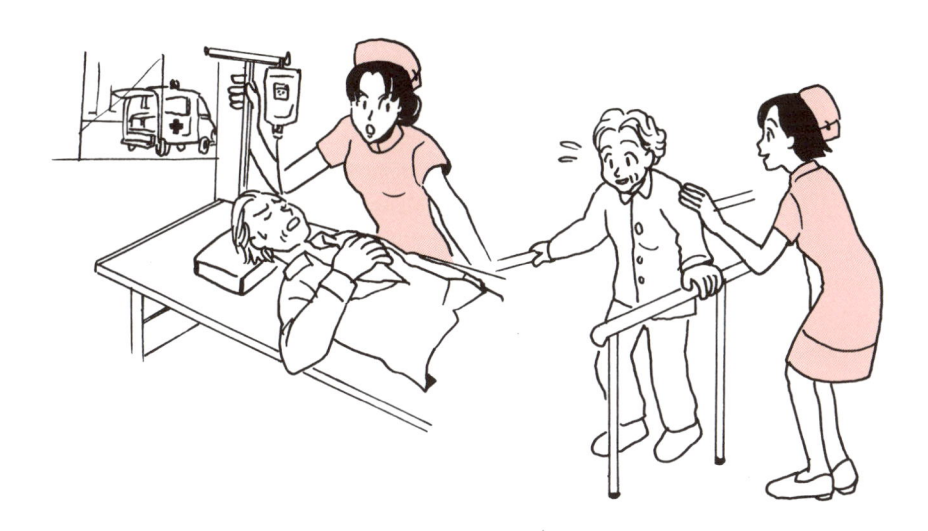

The majority of nurses work in hospitals. Many of these hospitals care for patients who are acutely ill. They also care for people who have accidents or need routine surgery. Other types of hospitals care for patients needing long-term treatment, rehabilitation or specialty care.

Many small hospitals provide all the needs of patients within the community. They have labor, delivery and nursery rooms; pediatric, surgical and medical units; and units for orthopedics or urology. These hospitals are often closely involved with the community. Usually the nurses for these hospitals also live in the community.

Some large hospitals have grown to meet the needs of

patients with special problems. These hospitals are often linked to medical schools in big cities. These hospitals usually have specialists and may care for patients from many different cities. The nurs-
15 es who work in these hospitals are also specialists. They work in intensive care units (ICU's) or in trauma units, or on transplant or dialysis teams. They may also specialize in very young patients or the elderly. These nurses often undergo further training and experience after their nursing programs to develop the knowledge and
20 skills needed to work in these specialized units.

Notes: 看護師のほとんどは病院で働く。
are acutely ill「急性の病気にかかっている」*cf.* chronic 慢性の (Chap.9)　**routine**「通常の」　**rehabilitation**「機能回復訓練」　**specialty care**「専門別医療」専門医が優秀な設備と人員を使って行う高度な医療。care は看護・介護だけでなく医療も意味する。**community**「地域社会」　**labor, delivery and nursery rooms**「陣痛室、分娩室、新生児室」陣痛室は分娩準備室とも言う。　**pediatric, surgical and medical units**「小児科、外科、内科」medical は '医学の' のほかに '内科の' も意味する。　**units for orthopedics or urology**「整形外科か泌尿器科」　**are closely involved with** *cf.* Chap. 5　**intensive care unit(s)**「集中治療室」　**trauma**「外傷」　**on transplant or dialysis teams**「移植チームや透析チームで」前置詞が in でなく on になっている点に注意。　**may also specialize in …**「…を専門にしていることもある」　**very young**「ひじょうに幼い」　**the elderly**「高齢者」　**nursing programs**「看護教育課程」

✚ Vocabulary

Match the similar expressions.

1. pediatrics　　（　）
2. orthopedics　（　）
3. urology　　　（　）
4. trauma　　　（　）
5. dialysis　　　（　）

a. method of treating kidney failure by removing wastes
b. physical or mental injury
c. department concerned with children
d. department concerned with urine
e. department concerned with putting bones straight

8. NURSES AND THE HOSPITAL

⊕ Questions & Answers

> 1. 2. Choose the best answer.
> 3. 4. Answer in English.
> 5. Make your own question.

1. What kind of treatment do hospitals give to "acutely" ill patients?
   a. long-term treatment   b. rehabilitation
   c. urgent treatment

2. What do many small hospitals offer?
   a. a variety of care services for patients in the community
   b. health care for patients from different cities
   c. specialty care for serious problems

3. What is a main difference between a small hospital in the community and a large hospital linked to a medical school?
   _____

4. Where do nursing specialists work?
   _____

5. Your question _____
   Answer _____

⊕ Grammar & Usage

> Fill in each blank with one word from the list below. Use each of them only once.

[for   in   of   to   with]

1. Many students live (   ) the dormitory near the hospital.
2. The patient (   ) breast cancer required round-the-clock nursing.
3. The large hospital linked (   ) the medical school is internationally famous.
4. Please take care (   ) the patient while I am away.
5. The hospital where Sue works does not have a unit (   ) terminal care.

2. So Busy Tonight

Dialogue A ⟨A: Nurse 1 B: Nurse 2 C: Patient D: Mother⟩

救急治療室で忙しく働きながら…。

A: The Emergency Room is so busy tonight. It seems everyone has come in today.

B: You said it! Will you take the blood pressure of that older woman who just sat down?

A: Fine. (To patient) I'd like to take your blood pressure now. Are you on any special medications or diet?

C: Yes. I take three pills for high blood pressure. But I ran out of them a week ago, so I haven't been taking anything.

A: Really? It's important to control your blood pressure so you don't have other problems.

D: Nurse, could you look at my little boy? He's coughing really hard. I don't think he can breathe.

A: Put him over here on this table. Let's see what's going on. I'm going to start some oxygen and notify the physician.

Notes: emergency room「救急治療室」 You said it!「全くその通り」 pill「丸薬」
run out of ～「～を切らす」 cough「咳をする」 notify ～「～に告げる」

Dialogue B ⟨A: Nurse Parker B: Nurse Brown C: Nursing Supervisor⟩

ICUで日直の看護師2人が多忙の中で…。

A: In the intensive care unit we're always busy. Both day and night. We never get to rest.	不平
B: I work 12 hours, all night—but get 4 days off each week.	応答
A: Here's the boss.	注意喚起
C: Nurse Brown, can you come back to the ward?	要請
B: Sure.	承諾
C: An elderly patient with Alzheimer's disease is confused and frightened. Maybe you can quiet her.	要請理由

Notes: ward「病棟，病室」 Alzheimer's disease「アルツハイマー病（老人性痴呆の一種）」
be confused「混乱している」

8. NURSES AND THE HOSPITAL

➕ True or False (Dialogue A)

Listen and write what you hear. Then circle T (true) or F (false).

1. _____ T / F
2. _____ T / F
3. _____ T / F
4. _____ T / F
5. _____ T / F

➕ Dialogue Practice (Dialogue B)

1. Substitute the words shown below.

▶ sentence: **Can you come back to the ward?**
   1. Will → _____
   2. Wouid → _____
   3. Could → _____
   4. the nurse station → _____

▶ sentence: **An elderly patient is confused and frightened.**
   1. I → _____
   2. We → _____
   3. relieved and satisfied → _____
   4. look → _____

2. Practice the dialogue.

➕ Vocabulary (Dialogues A and B)

Choose the word that means the same as the expression on the right, as it is used in the text.

1. emergency ( )   a. taking turns at working
2. pill   ( )   b. mixed up mentally
3. shift   ( )   c. small ball of solid medicine
4. ward   ( )   d. dangerous happening which must be dealt with at once
5. confused ( )   e. area in a hospital where patients sleep

3. LET'S TALK: Schedule and Work of the Nurse

✚ Schedule of the Day Nurse

Nurseは大体3交代制(three shifts)で働きます。あなたは見習いで、日勤のNurse、Patの働きぶりを見学したとしましょう。

1. ある時間帯の働きを示すcardが配られますから、その時間帯のPatの働きをよく読みましょう。
2. 他の時間帯のcardを持っている人と互いに質問しあい、Patの全体のscheduleを作ってみましょう。

	8:20
8:45	9:00
9:15	10:00
10:30	
	12:45
13:00	
14:00	16:00
16:30	16:45

3. 次の質問に答えましょう。

   1. What time did Pat start work and what was the first thing she did?
   2. What time did she have lunch and what time did the patients have lunch?
   3. When and how many times did she take the patients' temperature and blood pressure?
   4. How long was the nurses' meeting?
   5. How did she prepare patients to meet the doctors?

8. NURSES AND THE HOSPITAL

✚ Asking for and Giving Directions

次の語句を参考にしてパートナーと病院内の場所を聞きあいましょう。

1. 質問形式

   > Excuse me, where is the ....?

2. 答えに使える語句

It's on the first/second/third/fourth floor.	It's next to the staff room.
When you come out of the elevator, turn right.	It's opposite the shop.
Take the next corridor on the left.	It's between the X and the Y.
You will pass a telephone.	It's the third room on the right.

3. 聞く場所

   ### Student A

   > pediatrics ward   gynecology department
   > dermatology department   ENT department
   > casualty (emergency) department

   ### Student B

   > ophthalmology department   hematology department
   > ICU   X-ray department   geriatrics department

【病院地図】

1st floor

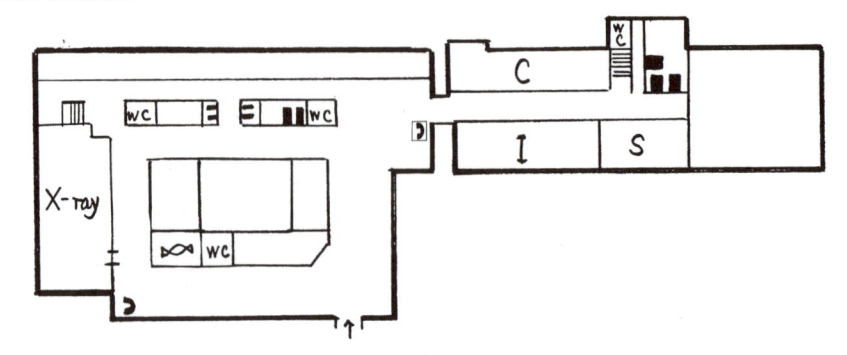

2nd floor

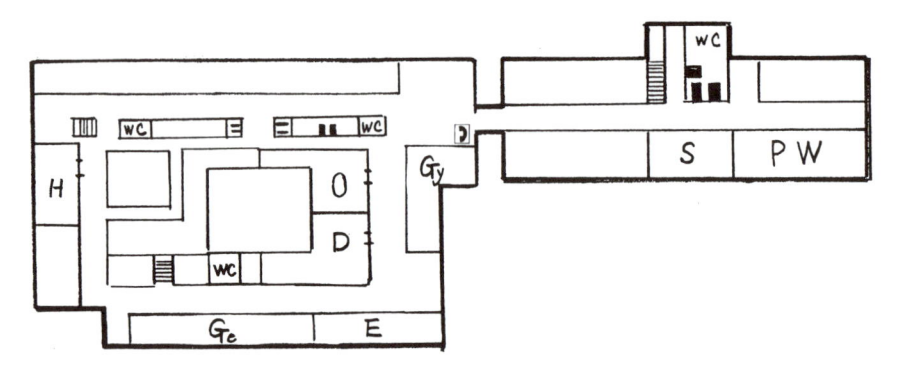

C: casualty (emergency) department （救急科）
D: dermatology department （皮膚科）
E: ENT（Ear Nose Throat） department （耳鼻咽喉科）
Ge: geriatrics department （老人病科）
Gy: gynecology department （婦人科）
H: hematology department （血液科）
I: intensive care unit （集中治療室）
PW: pediatrics ward （小児科病室）
O: ophthalmology department （眼科）
X-Ray: X-ray (radiology) department （レントゲン科）
S: staff room　　　　■■: elevator　　　　⋈: shop　　　　⌡: telephone

その他の科（department）
internal medicine （内科）　　surgery （外科）　　obstetrics （産科）
orthopedics （整形外科）　　urology （泌尿器科）　　neurology （神経科）
psychiatry （精神科）　　dentistry （歯科）

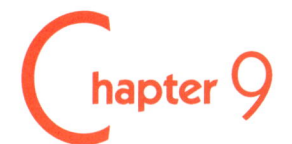

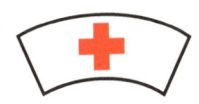

Chapter 9
NURSES IN THE COMMUNITY

1. Nurses Work Outside the Hospital

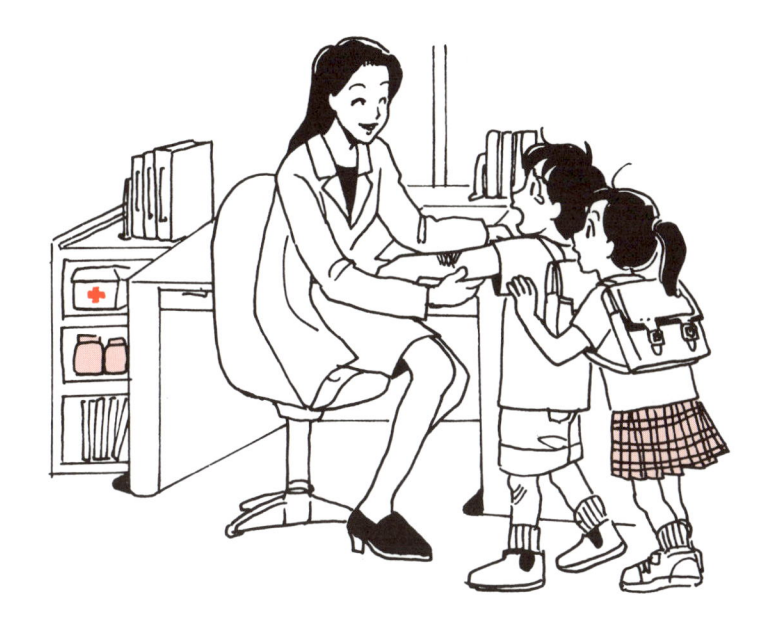

Nurses may work in a wide variety of places in the community. Employers have learned that nurses can help prevent employees from being injured on the job. Occupational health nurses may also develop programs for finding and treating patients with hypertension (high blood pressure), diabetes, lower back pain, or substance abuse problems. All of these problems may cause work loss if they go untreated.

Other nurses in the community go to patients' homes to help care for the ill. They often provide care so that the patients can stay at home and do not have to go to the hospital. They also teach the family how to care for the patient.

School nurses work in schools to treat minor health problems or injuries. Finding vision, hearing, or learning problems early helps prevent other problems from occurring later. Nurses also teach students about nutrition, hygiene, and safety.

Many nurses work with physicians in offices or clinics. They work with patients with only minor problems, or those who have chronic diseases. These nurses often spend time teaching patients about their diseases or medications. They provide information to help prevent healthy people from getting sick. They often work in universities, business offices, or health clubs to provide screening and educational programs. They may also staff AIDS or tuberculosis or women's health clinics.

Notes: **看護師は地域社会のさまざまな場所で働くことがある。**
prevent ... from 〜「…が〜するのを予防する」 **occupational health nurse(s)**「職業保健師」企業で働く人々の健康問題を扱う。 **develop programs**「計画を作る」 **lower back pain**「腰痛」 **substance abuse**「物質乱用」麻薬やアルコールの乱用のこと。 **work loss**「労働損失」 **go untreated**「治療されないままである、治療せずに放置される」 **school nurse(s)**「学校看護師、養護教諭」 **learning problems**「learning disability（学習障害）のこと」 **hygiene**「衛生」 **screening**「スクリーニング」ある特定の疾患（結核とか糖尿病とか）を見つけるために行う集団検診。 **educational programs** *cf.* Chap.2 **staff ...**「…の職員として働く」 **women's health clinic**「婦人科診療所」

🔴 Vocabulary

Match the similar expressions.

1. occupation ( )
2. abuse ( )
3. hygiene ( )
4. screening ( )
5. tuberculosis ( )

a. infectious disease especially in the lungs
b. cleanliness
c. examination to filter people
d. harmful misuse
e. job, employment

9. NURSES IN THE COMMUNITY

✚ Questions & Answers

> 1. 2. Choose the best answer.
> 3. 4. Answer in English.
> 5. Make your own question.

1. Why are occupational health nurses helpful to employers?
   a. They develop skills.   b. They prevent injury.
   c. They employ healthy workers.

2. What may happen if workers' health problems are neglected?
   a. It may reduce workers' efficiency.
   b. It may improve workers' efficiency.
   c. It may not change workers' efficiency.

3. What do nurses in the community do at patients' homes?
   _____
   _____

4. What do school nurses do?
   _____
   _____

5. Your question _____
   _____
   Answer _____

✚ Grammar & Usage

> Fill in each blank with one word from the list below. Use each of them only once.

[shall   will   can   would   may]

1. Ask me anything about your injury. I will do what I (   ).
2. Tom (   ) not succeed, because he has so many health problems.
3. (   ) you like another cup of tea?
4. I hope you (   ) get well and leave the hospital soon.
5. (   ) I open the window? You look sweaty.

2. To Prevent You from Getting Injured

Dialogue A ⟨A: Nurse   B: Manager⟩

工場でNurseが工場長を呼び止めて…。

A: Next week we'll start a series of programs here in the factory.

B: What will the programs be on?

A: One of the programs will be on how to make our factory safer. We've had several people injured recently because they didn't use equipment properly.

B: That should help prevent injuries.

A: Yes, and also, people who do the same job over and over—like work on the assembly line—often develop wrist injuries. We should be able to prevent them.

B: I hope all the workers can attend. It's a real problem for me when one of my staff is injured. All of us have to work harder then.

Notes: equipment「備品、装置」 assembly line「流れ作業列」

Dialogue B ⟨A: Nurse   B: Head Teacher⟩

学校でNurseが校長に相談して…。

A: It's time to schedule the students for their vision and hearing tests.	提言
B: Eh! I thought we'd already done that!	疑い
A: No, no. You're probably thinking of the scoliosis test.	否定, 指摘
B: Aah! Or maybe I'm thinking of last year's. Time passes so fast!	容認
A: Oh, by the way, Jenny Brown cut her elbow this morning. I gave her two stitches, put her arm in a sling and gave her some aspirin.	報告
B: What happened?	質問
A: She said that she slipped on the ice.	答え

Notes: scoliosis「(脊柱) 側湾 (症)」 elbow「ひじ」 stitch「(傷口を縫う) ひと針」 sling「つり包帯」

9. NURSES IN THE COMMUNITY

✚ True or False (Dialogue A)

Listen and write what you hear. Then circle T (true) or F (false).

1. _____ T / F
2. _____ T / F
3. _____ T / F
4. _____ T / F
5. _____ T / F

✚ Dialogue Practice (Dialogue B)

1. Substitute the words shown below.

▶ sentence: **It's time to schedule the tests.**
    1. sleep → _____
    2. take medicine → _____
    3. put on a gown → _____
    4. start the program → _____

▶ sentence: **I gave her two stitches.**
    1. him → _____
    2. an injection → _____
    3. some aspirin → _____
    4. 疑問文（you）→ _____

2. Practice the dialogue.

✚ Vocabulary (Dialogues A and B)

Choose the word that means the same as the expression on the right, as it is used in the text.

1. scoliosis (　)   a. joint where the arm bends
2. elbow   (　)   b. support for a damaged arm
3. stitch   (　)   c. curved shape of the spine
4. sling   (　)   d. medicine that lessens pain and fever
5. aspirin   (　)   e. thread for closing a wound

3. LET'S TALK: The Nurse Is Teaching Outside the Hospital

✚ Vocabulary

🎧74 1. イタリックの英語と日本語を結びましょう。CDを聴いて発音しましょう。

Do you prefer *diluted* or *concentrated* juice?	糖尿病
Have you ever *fed* bread to a duck?	冷蔵庫
Do you know anybody who has *diabetes*?	食べさせる
Do you store your vegetables in your *fridge* (*refrigerator*)?	薄めた
	濃縮した

2. 上の質問に答えましょう。パートナーと互いに質問しあいましょう。

🎧75 3. イタリックの英語と日本語を結びましょう。CDを聴いて発音しましょう。

1. The mother *weaned* her baby onto a *diet* of baby food.	血管
2. My baby has just started to eat *solid food*.	投薬量
3. She kept the baby food in cold *storage*.	ふく
4. The mother *encouraged* her good eating habits.	消毒薬
5. He gave her mother the prescribed *dosage* of insulin.	固形食
6. The nurse gave her a *hypodermic injection*.	引きぬく
7. The needle has not entered a *blood vessel*.	離乳する
8. The nurse *withdrew* the needle and *swabbed* the skin.	励ましてさせる
9. The nurse put some *antiseptic* on his cut.	食
	皮下注射
	貯蔵

9. NURSES IN THE COMMUNITY

76　4．CDをよく聴き、9つのワクチン(vaccine, vaccination)を発音してみましょう。

　　Diphtheria（ジフテリア）（　）　　Whooping cough（百日咳）（　）
　　Tetanus（破傷風）（　）　　　　　Polio（小児麻痺）（　）
　　Measles（麻疹）（　）　　　　　　Mumps（おたふく風邪）（　）
　　German Measles（風疹）（　）　　Meningitis（髄膜炎）（　）
　　Tuberculosis（結核）（　）

77　5．CDのDialogueをよく聴き、John（J）とMary（M）がどのワクチンを受けたことがあるか上の表に印をつけましょう。

6．今までにどんなワクチンを受けたことがあるか、パートナーと互いに質問しあいましょう。

　　問：Have you had a *hepatitis*（肝炎）vaccination?
　　　　　　　　　　　　　　　　　　　　　（イタリックの部分をかえてみる。）

✚ Role Play

> 設定：訪問看護師(nurse)と介護者(carer)との会話です。介護者は赤ちゃんを育てるかたわら、糖尿病の母の介護もしています。従って赤ちゃんの食事やワクチン、母の食事やインスリン注射について、Nurseにいろいろたずねたいと思っています。

[Role Playの方法]
1．クラスを9～10人ずつのグループに分け、さらに4～5人ずつに分け、一方をNurseグループ、他方をCarerグループとします。
2．グループ内の人は各々違うCarer Task Cardをもらいます。また、それぞれのCarer Task Cardの右下に小さく書いてある記号のNurse Role Cardももらいます。
3．まず自分の役割のCardをよく読み、内容を相手に言うことができるようにしましょう。

4. Nurse 役の人は、次々に家を訪問するつもりで Carer の質問に答えましょう。たとえば次のように会話を始めます。

> Hi, I'm Nurse Penny. How are you today?
> I've come to see if you have any questions about (weaning your baby.)

Carer 役の人は、次に自分がなる記号の Nurse 以外の Nurse から家族の介護について情報を得るようにします。

5. Carer 役の人が Nurse 役の人達から必要な情報すべてを得ることができたら、役割をかえて同様にしてみましょう。

6. 両方の役割をやり終えたら、答を持ちよって皆で次の質問に答えましょう。

1. Why does the baby cry after you give it a concentrated mixture?

2. When might the baby be ready to eat solid food?

3. Is it a good idea to give it food just to stop it crying? Why or why not?

4. What vaccinations does the one-year-old baby need?

5. What vaccinations will the two-month-old baby need soon?

6. Does the 4-year-old child need a tuberculosis vaccination soon?

7. Explain the first three steps of giving a hypodermic injection.

8. How should you store insulin?

9. In what dosage and how often should you give insulin?

10. What diet is suitable for a person with diabetes?

Chapter 10

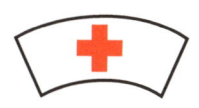

NURSING IN THE FUTURE

1. How Will Nursing Change in the Future?

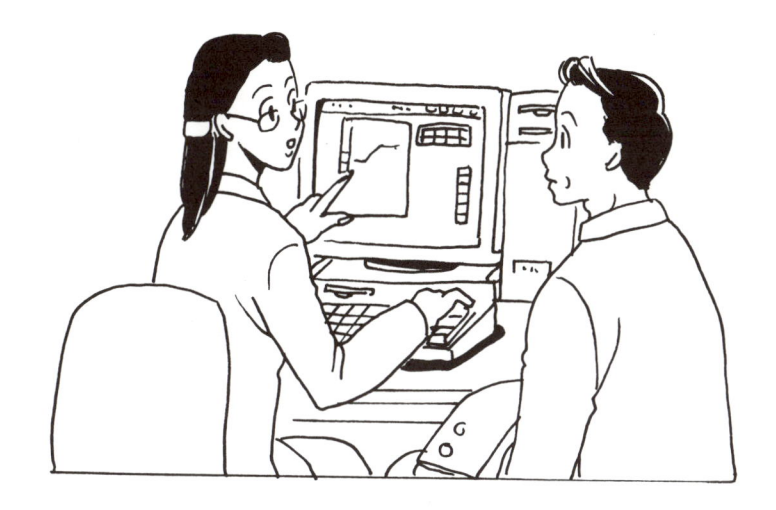

New technology has given nurses equipment to help them care for patients. This has forced nurses to learn and understand many new things. What will play the biggest role in reshaping nursing? Information technology, genetic engineering, medical ethics, virtual reality or transplantation?

The dramatic increase in knowledge is certain to continue. The Internet has made it easier to notice changes in what nurses need to know, how to find it, and what they may legally do. In the future, nurses may use computers to advise, counsel and educate patients. Many new laws may arise to protect the nurse, the patient-nurse relationship, and patient records. Thus, there may be a redefinition of who nurses are and what they contribute to patient care.

In the future, nurses may continue to develop direct care specialties in nursing. Some nurses may work more with acutely ill patients in hospitals, while other nurses may provide primary care to patients in the community. Many nurses will do research to help them practice more scientifically. While continuing to work with physicians, nurses will work more independently as they gain more knowledge and as the demands for health care services increase.

Notes: 新しい科学技術は看護師に患者さんの看護を助ける機器を与えてくれた。
reshaping …＜ reshape …「…を作り直す」 **information technology**「情報工学」 **genetic engineering**「遺伝子工学」gene [dʒíːn] が遺伝子。 **changes in …**「…における変化」change の後には前置詞 in が来ることが多い。（例）a change in the weather 天候の変化。 **patient record(s)**「患者記録」看護師がつける公的な記録。nurse's record「看護記録」とも言う。 **redefinition**「再定義。定義のし直し」 **direct care**「直接看護」排泄、運動、清潔など患者に直接かかわる看護のこと。連絡、記録、物品管理などの間接看護に対する。 **primary care**「一次医療」患者に最初に接触する医師・看護師などによる医療。 **practice**「実践する」 **health care services**「医療サービス」

✚ Vocabulary

Match the similar expressions.

1. equipment   (　)   a. earliest
2. ethics   (　)   b. network of computer links
3. transplantation (　)   c. moving an organ from one
4. the Internet   (　)   person to another
5. primary   (　)   d. science which deals with
                              morals
                           e. things needed to do something

10. NURSING IN THE FUTURE

✛ Questions & Answers

> 1. 2. Choose the best answer.
> 3. 4. Answer in English.
> 5. Make your own question.

1. What will nurses do in the future?
   a. They will care for fewer patients in the community.
   b. They will work harder and longer in hospitals.
   c. They will use more advanced technology.

2. What helps nurses deal with the increase of knowledge?
   a. e-mail   b. the Internet   c. virtual reality

3. For what could nurses use computers?
   _____
   _____

4. What could new laws do for nurses?
   _____
   _____

5. Your question _____
   _____
   Answer _____

✛ Grammar & Usage

> Write the correct verb tense.

1. The hospital closes at 6 o'clock. You (   ) in time if you hurry. [be]
2. Only a few people (   ) mechanical things when our company was started up. [understand]
3. They (   ) their work by the time their boss comes back. [finish]
4. The patient (   ) from a breathing problem since he entered this hospital. [suffer]
5. Don't worry. You (   ) better after this medicine. [feel]

2. Nursing on the Internet

Dialogue A 〈A and B: Nurses〉

これからのNurseの仕事を話しあって…。

A: I've taken a job with the United Health Care System.

B: What are you going to do?

A: I'm going to teach a series of classes on the Internet for patients with diabetes in four different states.

B: I didn't know you could legally do that.

A: Yes, I just received my national nursing license that allows me to practice throughout the country, not just in one state.

B: Aren't you worried about some patients in the class learning about problems of other patients?

A: No, the class is set up so I can talk with everyone, but what the patient says to me is confidential. No one else can hear what they say.

B: That really sounds exciting.

Notes:　state「(アメリカ合衆国の) 州」　legally「合法的に」　confidential「内密の」

Dialogue B 〈A: Student Nurse, B: Teacher〉

看護学生と先生が未来を語って…。未来は本当にバラ色かしら？

A: Nowadays everybody uses computers. What do you think will happen in the future?	導入質問
B: Well, virtual reality is becoming more and more popular and robots will become more powerful.	答え
A: And will robots perform operations?	質問
B: Actually, some do now! The biggest change will be in genetic engineering. I read that they could soon grow human body parts in genetically-engineered, cloned animals.	答え　他の例提示
A: Yes, but there'll also be new problems in the future. For example, there's been a 50% drop in male fertility over the last ten years.	問題強調

Notes:　cloned「無性的につくられた」　fertility「受精能力」

10. NURSING IN THE FUTURE

✚ True or False (Dialogue A)

Listen and write what you hear. Then circle T (true) or F (false).

1. _____ T / F
2. _____ T / F
3. _____ T / F
4. _____ T / F
5. _____ T / F

✚ Dialogue Practice (Dialogue B)

1. Substitute the words shown below or follow the instructions.

▶ sentence: **What do you think will happen in the future?**
   1. is wrong with him → _____
   2. happened to him → _____
   3. we should give him → _____
   4. about smoking → _____

▶ sentence: **There'll be new problems in the future.**
   1. improvements → _____
   2. a 25% drop → _____
   3. 否定文 → _____
   4. 疑問文 → _____

2. Practice the dialogue.

✚ Vocabulary (Dialogues A and B)

Choose the word that means the same as the expression on the right, as it is used in the text.

1. confidential ( )   a. allowed by law
2. legal   ( )   b. nonsexually-produced
3. genetic   ( )   c. being able to reproduce
4. cloned   ( )   d. of substances passed on in the
                            cells from the parents
5. fertile   ( )   e. to be kept secret

3. LET'S TALK: What Type of Nurse Do You Want to Be?

✚ Vocabulary

1. イタリックの単語を下の同じ意味の日本語の(　)内に書き入れましょう。

   1. An *anesthetist* is a doctor who makes the patient sleep.
   2. To *make the rounds* means to visit all the patients in the ward.
   3. A woman who is *pregnant* has a baby growing inside her.
   4. To *diagnose* means to discover and identify an illness.
   5. *Vital signs* are temperature, pulse, respiration and blood pressure.
   6. A *sterilized* object, such as a contact lens, has been cleaned.
   7. A *surgeon* is a doctor who does operations.
   8. To *monitor* is to observe something for a long time.
   9. *First aid treatment* is the medical help you give to someone very quickly when they have an accident.
   10. To *scrub* is to clean your hands before an operation
   11. A *G.P.*(*general practitioner*) is a family doctor.

   外科医　　　　　　　　　　　(　　　　　　　)
   妊娠している　　　　　　　　(　　　　　　　)
   (手術前に) ごしごし手を洗う　(　　　　　　　)
   一般開業医　　　　　　　　　(　　　　　　　)
   回診する　　　　　　　　　　(　　　　　　　)
   生命徴候　　　　　　　　　　(　　　　　　　)
   滅菌した　　　　　　　　　　(　　　　　　　)
   麻酔医　　　　　　　　　　　(　　　　　　　)
   応急処置　　　　　　　　　　(　　　　　　　)
   監視する　　　　　　　　　　(　　　　　　　)
   診断する　　　　　　　　　　(　　　　　　　)

2. CDを聴いて発音しましょう。

10. NURSING IN THE FUTURE

✚ Dialogue Practice

1. Dialogueを読んで空所に適当な語を入れてみましょう。
2. CDを聴いて確かめましょう。
3. パートナーと練習してみましょう。

Dialogue 〈A: Friend B: Trainee Nurse（研修中のナース）〉

研修中のNurseが友達と出会って…。

A: So what type of nurse do you want to be?

B: Now I'm training as a general nurse. I want to be *an occupational health nurse* later.

A: _____?

B: Well, *they work in companies. They look after the workers. They try to prevent the workers from becoming ill.*

A: _____?

B: *They* also *give first aid treatment.*

✚ Role Play

どんなNurseになりたいか、そのNurseはどんなことをするか、互いに聞きあいましょう。

[Role Playの方法]

1. あなたがなりたいNurseのカードをよく読んで、3つのjob（仕事）の内容を覚えましょう。
2. Dialogue Practiceのなかのイタリック部分をあなたのものにかえて、パートナーと会話してみましょう。
    注：Trainee Nurse役の人は、仕事の内容を聞かれたら最初に2つ答え、次に残りの1つを答えます。また、Friend役の人は、パートナーが言っていることがわからない場合、たとえばWhat does that mean?と言って説明を求めましょう。**Vocabulary**を参考にしてください。
3. 役割をかえて同様にしてみましょう。
4. 違う番号のNurseになりたいパートナーを見つけて、同じように会話してみましょう。

5. 6種類全部のNurseの仕事がわかったら、次の質問に対する答えを選んで番号で答えましょう。

1. What do midwives do? _____
2. What do head nurses do? _____
3. What do family clinic nurses do? _____
4. What do scrub nurses do? _____
5. What do nurse anesthetists do? _____
6. What do visiting nurses do? _____

答

1. They help women through childbirth.
2. They count the tools before and after the operation.
3. They order equipment and drugs.
4. They give medication to patients at home.
5. They prepare patients to meet the doctor.
6. They weigh and wash the newborn babies.
7. They assist a patient when he or she comes around.
8. They pass (give) the sterilized tools to the surgeon.
9. They visit sick people in their home.
10. They arrange the nurses' timetables.
11. They lift (move) the patient onto the operating table.
12. They advise pregnant women about their diet.

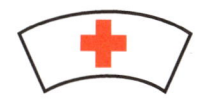

Useful Expressions

> **Dialogue B**

Chapter 1 : 痛そうですね

　　　It looks like your wrist is hurting you.（間接的な質問）

　　　Have you sprained it?（直接的な質問）

　　　Maybe you should give it a rest every couple of hours.（示唆）

Chapter 2 : ほんとにそうね

　　　It's important to observe the patient.（例の提示）

　　　We must write down what the patient does.（例の提示）

　　　That's true. Definitely.（同意）

Chapter 3 : 大丈夫ですよ

　　　I've had diabetes for a long long time.（患者の状況）

　　　The insulin will help you.（安心させる）

　　　Don't worry about that.（安心させる）

Chapter 4 : 見せてちょうだい

　　　Let's see how heavy you are! Just stand on here.（要請、命令）

　　　Can I see your teeth? Show me your teeth.（要請、命令）

Chapter 5 : どうなんでしょうか

　　　Can you tell me how Jeremy is?（問いかけ）

　　　We're going to give him a transfusion.（これからの予定）

Chapter 6 : こんなことがあるんですが

　　　Mr. Black said that he's allergic to penicillin.（情報提供）

　　　How much should I give him？（指示をあおぐ）

Chapter 7 : こんなことがありました

 She complained of nausea.（報告）

 Blood tests showed that she had high levels of digitalis.（検査の結果報告）

Chapter 8 : 来てくれますか

 Can you come back to the ward ?（要請）

 An elderly patient with Alzheimer's disease is confused and frightened.（状況説明）

Chapter 9 : そろそろする時ですね

 It's time to schedule the students for their vision and hearing tests.（提言）

 I gave her two stitches.（報告）

 What happened?（質問）

Chapter 10 : どんなになると思う？

 What do you think will happen in the future?（導入質問）

 There'll also be new problems in the future.（問題も強調）

LET'S TALK

Chapter 1 : ～しています（ナースの仕事）

 A nurse is feeding a patient.

 When was the last time you went to the hospital?

Chapter 2 : ～に使われます（看護機器）

 It's a machine.

 It's made of wood.

 It's used for eating.

Chapter 3 : お聞きしたいのですが（患者への質問）

 I'd like to ask you a few questions about your personal details.

Is there anything else you want?
Is there any food which you don't like?

Chapter 4 : どうしましたか（患者への質問）
What happened?
When did it happen?
Where did it happen?
How did the speaker feel?

Chapter 5 : どうすればいいかしら（困ったことの対処）
What do you think is the problem?
I think that the bed's too short for the patient.
I agree. That's a good idea.
How are you? I'm sorry. Anything else I can do? Certainly.

Chapter 6 : どうしたらいいでしょうか（医師に相談する）
How should I lower the temperature?
Can I use a catheter to measure urine?

Chapter 7 : どの科にかかればいいかしら（科をたずねる）
What do you call a doctor who specializes in hematology?
In which department do hematologists work?

Chapter 8 : どこですか（病院勤務、病院案内）
Excuse me, where is the pediatrics ward?

Chapter 9 : 聞きたいことはありませんか（訪問看護）
I've come to see if you have any questions about weaning your baby.

Chapter 10 : どんなナースになりたい？（将来像）
What type of nurse do you want to be?
What do they do?

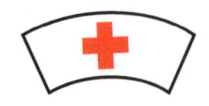

Parts and Organs of the Body

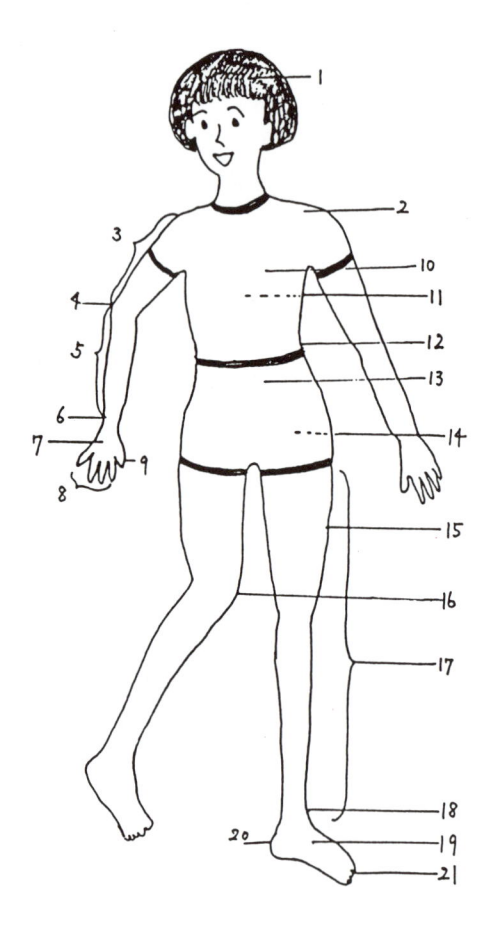

Parts

1. head   2. shoulder   3. upper arm
4. elbow   5. forearm   6. wrist
7. hand   8. finger   9. thumb
10. chest   11. back   12. waist
13. abdomen（腹）   14. buttock（尻）
15. thigh（もも）   16. knee
17. leg   18. ankle   19. foot
20. heel   21. toe

Organs

1. trachea（気管）
2. esophagus（食道）
3. lung（肺）   4. heart（心臓）
5. liver（肝臓）   6. stomach（胃）
7. pancreas（膵臓）   8. kidney（腎臓）
9. small intestine（小腸）
10. large intestine（大腸）
11. rectum（直腸）   12. bladder（膀胱）

著作権法上、無断複写・複製は禁じられています。

English for Nursing Students   [B-312]
看護系学生のための総合英語

改装 1 刷	2005年4月 5日
改装 16 刷	2021年4月10日

著　者	Marilyh W. Edmunds, Paul Price
	大瀧　祥子　Sachiko Ohtaki　引地　岳雄　Takeo Hikichi
発行者	南雲　一範　Kazunori Nagumo
発行所	株式会社　南雲堂
	〒162-0801　東京都新宿区山吹町361
	NAN'UN-DO Publishing Co., Ltd.
	361 Yamabuki-cho, Shinjuku-ku, Tokyo 162-0801, Japan
	振替口座：00160-0-46863
	TEL: 03-3268-2311（代表）/ FAX: 03-3269-2486
	編集者　TA / RO
製版所	SOUTH FLIGHT
装　丁	Nスタジオ
検　印	省　略
コード	ISBN4-523-17312-5　C0082

Printed in Japan

E-mail　nanundo@post.email.ne.jp
URL　　https://www.nanun-do.co.jp/

CD付き ECCが贈る 最強の英検対策

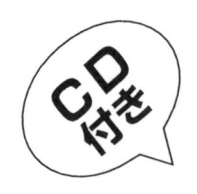

リニューアル英検 完全対応シリーズ

10日間完成　英検準1級一次試験対策
10日間完成　英検 2 級 一次試験対策
10日間完成　英検準2級一次試験対策
10日間完成　英検 3 級 一次試験対策

ECC編　A5判並製　定価（本体1600円＋税）

最新出題傾向に合わせ、ECCが総力を結集して研究したオリジナル問題を収録。短期間で自分の弱点を発見、補強し、オールラウンドな英語力がつくように構成。英検一次試験対策には格好の問題集。

7日間完成　英検準1級二次試験対策
7日間完成　英検 2 級 二次試験対策
7日間完成　英検準2級二次試験対策
7日間完成　英検 3 級 二次試験対策

ECC編　A5判並製　定価（本体1500円＋税）

英検二次試験の面接問題にターゲットを絞った教材。面接で多く用いられる題材を取り上げ、丁寧な解説をつけた。付属のCDを使いながらリスニング力を上げつつ、本番さながらの試験を体験できる。